Every
Step
Counts

Every
Step
Counts

ADRIAN BESLEY

CARLTON
BOOKS

Published in 2005

10 9 8 7 6 5 4 3 2 1

A CIP catalogue record for this book is available from the British Library.

ISBN 1-84442-360-3

Editor: Nigel Matheson
Typesetting: E-type, Liverpool
Project Art Direction: Luke Griffin
Production: Lisa French
Printed in China

Contents

Introduction

This book is designed to be used in conjunction with a pedometer and comes complete with instructions on how to use it most effectively. This clever little gadget gives you the ability to set yourself measurable goals, as well as helping you plot your progress from day to day, and from week to week.

The pedometer, which keeps a running total of every step you take, is vital to show you how you are getting on and to help you maintain your resolve to see the programme though.

The pages that follow will explain exactly why walking can be so beneficial for you and they also contain a low-impact fitness and weight-loss programme, which is based on reaching the magical 10,000 step per day mark recommended by health foundations across the world.

This book is all about setting yourself targets and achieving them. Regular walking is the easy way to get fit and lose weight and there's no need to join an expensive gym or completely transform your regular lifestyle.

Finally, remember one thing: the more steps you do, the more benefits you will see to your fitness and waistline.

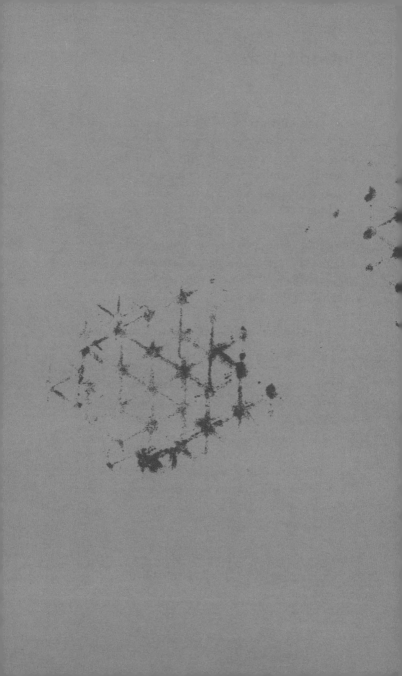

1 Welcome to the World of Walking!

You're on your way! By buying this book, you've joined the millions around the world who are ready to get on the move for their health. This is a programme with no expensive fitness club fees, no embarrassing leotards or crop tops and no painful exhortations to follow the body-contorting moves of the latest size-eight soap star. All you need to start improving your fitness is the pedometer, a comfortable pair of shoes and a modicum of will power.

The vast majority of us lead sedentary lives – sitting behind computers all day and slumped on the sofa after work. We might walk the children to school, amble to the bus stop and pop round to the sandwich shop at lunchtime, but that's the extent of our exercise. Even the thought of an aerobics class or an hour in the gym brings us out in a sweat. But just through walking a little extra, every day, we can make changes in our fitness that will produce a difference in our health, our waistlines and our whole outlook on life.

The pedometer simply counts each stride you make until you reset it. When we know how many steps we are taking a day or a week, we can set ourselves realistic goals and objectives to increase our physical activity. Even better, by measuring our stride, it can enable us to work out how far we have walked and how many calories we may have burned. All this from a little box! OK, it won't get you out of bed on a winter's morning; it won't make you get off the bus a stop early or put your coat on for a lunchtime stroll. That's down to you – but having that box might just supply the incentive to get you to the magic 10,000-step mark.

This book also aims to help you. It will give you ideas for notching up those extra steps and tips on fitting them into a busy day. It will offer you hints on how to walk effectively (and you thought you'd been doing it since you were very young!) and how to beat the walker's blues – giving you a friendly nudge on those days when you just can't be bothered. It puts your newfound fitness into the context of an all-round healthy lifestyle.

As well as being the perfect accessory to help you become more healthy, the pedometer can also be a great aid in helping you lose weight. The book will reveal how developing your step count in line with a sensible diet can aid weight loss, but the great part is that you set your own goals and your own pace. Whatever your personal objectives, you will find the fill-in pages a perfect way to set targets, record your progress and even compare your achievements with the real-life case studies which follow.

TOP TIP

Your walking shoes should be replaced about every 500 miles.

However, before you begin, remember this is still *exercise* and without proper prior consideration it is possible to harm your health. Do you have a heart condition, asthma or any other condition that could be exacerbated? Do you have knee, ankle, foot or other physical weaknesses that might prevent you from increasing your daily steps? And, are you aware of your general fitness level and your capacity for taking on more exercise? If you have any doubts whatsoever, consult your doctor before changing your everyday routine.

Regardless of your fitness level, throughout your walking programme, make sure your increments are manageable before undertaking them and be aware of what your body is telling you. You are not obliged to feel any burn, and you definitely do not have to "walk 'til you drop". You may feel mildly and pleasantly tired and your heartbeat may quicken a little, but this is not a programme in which you need to feel exhausted or which should cause any part of your body to ache. If you feel any physical pain or breathlessness, be sure to stop immediately and rest.

Many of those who have taken to walking with a pedometer have soon realized what pleasure can be had in a simple walk. You notice so many aspects of your environment that pass by unnoticed in the claustrophobic interiors of cars and public transport; you notice that your mind feels uncluttered, much more able to focus on resolving problems or planning activities and it is quite possible that, like many others, you will find yourself much more at ease with yourself and with people you encounter in life.

Did You Know?

Walking burns approximately the same amount of calories per mile as running, but delivers only one quarter of the jolts to your muscles and joints.

CASE STUDIES which show how regular walking can change your life.

Driving the point home
Sasha, graphic designer – aged 30

It came as quite a shock to Sasha when she discovered her busy office job was only providing a maximum of 3,500 steps during the workday. Despite a sterling attempt to make more tea for her colleagues, to visit friends in other departments and to collect everyone else's printing, she still wasn't nudging up her total significantly.

Her salvation came as she was driving to work one morning. Taking a corner too fast she dumped her car in a ditch – fortunately emerging unscathed. Forced to live a vehicle-less life, Sasha suddenly found the answer: a long walk to and from the station, a change of underground trains and another brisk stroll to the office were adding an amazing 3,000 steps to her tally. Seeing the magic 10,000 was now in sight galvanized her into more action. She coerced different friends into taking lunchtime walks, went on foot instead of getting the train and, of course, no longer had the car for her evening trips to the cinema, restaurants or the launderette.

"I always thought my car was an essential part of my life," she says. "Even when I was trying to figure out how to get more steps into my day, I hadn't considered leaving it behind. Shortly after it was repaired, I sold it and haven't looked back."

Doggedly determined

Kim, housewife and mother – aged 41

Mother of three, Kim knew it was going to be difficult, but she was determined to regain the fitness she once took for granted. "I wasn't really keen to go to a gym or join an exercise class," says the 41-year-old. "Spending valuable time with my family was the priority for me, but I still needed a way of staying healthy that I could incorporate into an already busy lifestyle." Walking the children back and forth between school and her daily chores meant Kim was already notching up a good few thousand steps, but to make the jump to 10,000 was proving more tricky. "Whenever I decided I'd take a walk, there always seemed something more urgent to do," she recalls. Then along came Roger. "It was the children's idea, but I fell in love with him straight away," Kim confesses. Roger, a rescue dog with a fair amount of Labrador in him, was one bundle of canine energy. Suddenly, Kim found herself having to take Roger out for a good walk at least twice a day – and she loved it. "Without trying, I found I was doing eight or nine thousand steps a day and felt fitter than I had in years."

From fast food to fast feet

Steve, logistics co-ordinator – aged 52

The most exercise Steve ever got was pushing his chair across the office to get to the printer. Since his thirties, Steve had let himself go, quit the little sport he did and settled in to a life of fatty food and beer. As Steve's weight crept up and up, he realised something had to be done. "I read the books and started trying diets, but even if I stuck to them for a while, they never seemed to work." Then a friend gave him a pedometer. "I always hated walking, but suddenly there seemed a point – I just loved seeing that counter go up and up. At first I enjoyed my evening walks and noticed I was even losing weight. But as the nights got colder, the pub looked ever more tempting."

As his weight crept back, it seemed Steve would give up. Then a friend introduced him to the treadmill at the gym. "It was perfect. I was able to adjust the speed and gradient, and keep an eye on the distance I had walked.
It gave me a whole new incentive to carry on."

> **TOP TIP**
>
> Set your alarm for 30 minutes earlier in the morning and then you can fit in another 1,000 steps.

Group practice

Maureen, pensioner – aged 67

Maureen hadn't wanted to go to the community centre. She hadn't felt like doing much for weeks. "I'd just sit in my chair, wondering whether to make a cup of tea and usually deciding not to bother," she confesses. But it was at the centre that she read about the launch of a healthy walks scheme.

"I just felt I had to do something to get myself out of the mire," she recalls. The first walk was cold, wet and miserable, but once the organiser told her about the pedometer, she knew she would be back. Over two years later, she takes long walks nearly every day and joins the group every Thursday.

"I've made so many new friends," she says. "The more I walked, the more confident and clear-minded I felt. I even lost weight."

Maureen is now an organizer herself, but she'll never forget her first walk.

When good neighbours become good friends

Rhoda, mother and housewife – aged 48

Rhoda has had to battle against her weight all her life. In her mid-twenties, she had lost over eight stone (112 lbs) on a diet that had taken all her effort. Now, 25 years later, the weight had crept back on. "Not only did I feel depressed, but it made me less inclined to exercise – I felt powerless against an ever-increasing waistline." It was her neighbou's idea to start using the pedometer. "I think it brought out my competitive spirit," she admits. "I was quite a fierce netball player in my schooldays."

The friends began taking walks together and comparing totals, swapping hints and congratulating each other even if they secretly hoped their tally would be the highest.

"We really spurred each other on. If I spied her walking round the garden, I'd take a few turns around the house. It wasn't like dieting; it was fun and we'd share a lot of laughs about our experiences."

Rhoda once again began to lose weight and even though her neighbour eventually moved away has kept on walking. "I still ring her up and ask her how many steps she's done today," says Rhoda. "And I still get a buzz if I've done a few more!"

All in a week's work

Vicky and Lee, clerical workers – aged 28

Vicky and her boyfriend Lee took up the 10,000-step challenge together. Both office workers, they needed to think hard of ways of increasing their tally. "We both did what we could," Vicky insists. "We walked instead of driving to the station, took a stroll at lunchtimes and we'd meet up after work for a walk to a restaurant, an exhibition or the cinema."

But, most days, when they came to look at the pedometer their tallies would be little over 7,000. Then, one weekend away, they joined friends on their Sunday afternoon stroll. "Four hours it took us," Lee recalls. "We were both exhausted, but we'd really enjoyed it, and we realized we'd taken nearly 20,000 steps."

As their weekend expedition became a regular occurrence, they started keeping a weekly rather than a daily tally. "We get really excited about it now," says Vicky. "Getting out maps and planning our route – and trying to make sure we finish the week with our pedometers reading a magic 70,000!"

Variety – the steps of life

Kate, dental technician – aged 24

Kate started using a pedometer after she had given up her gym membership. "It was costing me too much and I was getting pretty bored of the same old faces and equipment." Not that she took to the walking that easily. "I couldn't believe the effort involved. I'm an active person and I thought I'd notch them up in a flash," she says. Actually, Kate was determined and kept going by constantly changing her routine. "I have a choice of walks depending on my mood," she says, having kept up her walking for almost a year. "Sometimes it's the shopping centre; it's amazing how many steps you can do, if you do all three levels. Sometimes I'll go to the athletic track and try to speed-walk some laps or, if I can persuade them, I'll just grab a girlfriend and spend an hour strolling around having a good gossip."

Wherever Kate's walking now, it's not going to be back to those dreary nights at the gym.

DID YOU KNOW

The average person walks the equivalent of three and a half times around the earth in a lifetime.

Stepping out at suppertime

Shirley, working mother – 41-year-old

Busy in a solicitor's office and tending to three children under five, Shirley was not surprised to discover that she was only taking 2,500 steps a day. "I was either bogged down in the office or stuck with children who couldn't or wouldn't walk far," she says. "No amount of trips to the photocopier or the office kettle was going to help get my total near 10,000." But Shirley was nothing if not determined. "I vowed I would get there so, come storm or snow, as soon as the kids were in bed, I was into my old raincoat and off down the street. I worked out a three-mile circular walk and did it every evening – while my partner cooked dinner!" Over a relatively short period of time, Shirley's friends began to comment on how her shape had changed. She lost a little weight, but her hips, waist and thighs were all smaller. And she noticed other changes. "I soon began to notice how I felt fitter, how much calmer I was at work and home and how I enjoyed my walks so much. I'd dread missing out on one."

Top Walking Tips

- Get a friend or a partner to join you – like most things, it's better with two!
- Leave the car in the garage – tell yourself it's only for trips over five miles.
- Have one regular 20-minute (or even longer) walk a day.
- Join a walking club – ask at the library or the local council for your nearest group.
- Build a brisk 10-minute walk in the morning and afternoon into your daily schedule.
- Take up a "walking" sport like golf, bowls or 10-pin bowling.
- Use telephone time – pace the floor when you are on a hands-free phone at home or work.
- Always choose the parking bay furthest away from the shops.
- Get a dog – it'll need walking at least twice a day and some working dogs need a good few miles each day.
- Visit an athletics track and work on your 400-metre personal best.

Get your steps in... at home:

- Walk on the spot for five or 10 minutes when you get up – exercise you can do in your pyjamas!
- Make the most of chores – walk on the spot while washing up and ironing.

- Ditch the remote – that's 10 steps every time you change the channel on the TV.
- Work out a minute's route around the house or garden and take it whenever you can.
- Put the radio or some music on and dance your way through a couple of hundred steps.
- Step your way through your favourite half-hour comedy.
- Get up and walk around every time there is a commercial break on TV.
- Rather than sitting waiting for your favourite programme to start, take yourself on a timed walk.
- Cut the grass, or clean the car or the outside of your windows.
- Get out and do some pottering and weeding in the garden – the plants will see the benefit as well.
- Get your steps in… on the streets
- Leave the car at home and use public transport and foot power.
- Pretend you have won the lottery and take yourself window shopping.
- Walk to the supermarket and get a taxi or a bus home with your weekly shop.
- Do a couple of laps of the supermarket aisles before you start shopping – you might even spot a bargain.
- Get a job as a professional dog-walker and earn money for your steps!
- Get your husband, children or parents out for a walk with you – you'll find you are closer than ever.
- Take an interest in local history and do some exploring around the area where you live.

- Get a newspaper or pizza leaflet delivery round – more cash for your Christmas fund!
- If you stop for petrol, walk home and let your partner drive the car back.
- If you have to wait for prescriptions, or repairs, or to see a doctor – fill the time by taking a short circular walk where you can.

DID YOU KNOW?

Only three out of 10 people do enough exercise, but eight out of 10 think they do.

Get your steps in... in the working day

- Get up half an hour early and get in some extra steps. It'll set you up nicely for a high-achieving day.
- Walk to the next station, a few bus stops along the route or even all the way – you'll be saving money, too.
- If you drive to work, leave the car a good ten minutes or more away from your workplace. You'll be up for the walk in the morning and have no choice by the evening!
- Don't email anything or send anything internally that you can deliver on foot. That personal touch might do your career some good as well.
- Volunteer to go out and get the coffees.
- If smokers take a break, take one too and nip off for a five-minute stroll.
- If you are kept waiting for a meeting – find a short loop you can walk until they are ready. If there are two or three of you, suggest a walking meeting. You'll find you all think more clearly with less verbal rambling when you are on your feet.
- Plan your lunchtime walk to maximize your time. Buy your lunch on the way and eat it when you get back, if you can.
- If you are socializing after work, arrange to meet somewhere you can reach on foot.
- Make a routine of taking an evening walk a couple of hours after your meal.

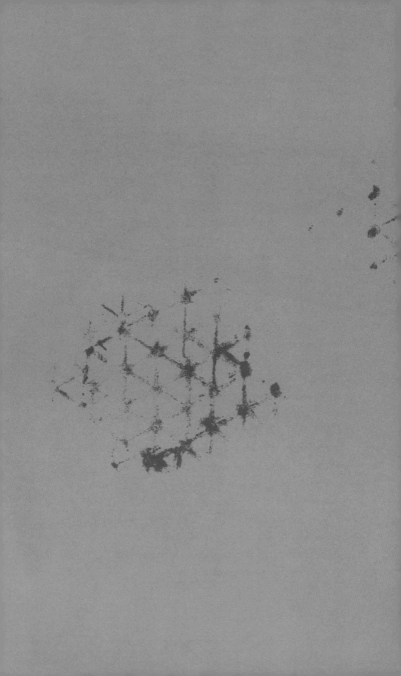

2 Introducing the Pedometer

"THE SUM OF THE WHOLE IS THIS: WALK AND BE HAPPY; WALK AND BE HEALTHY. THE BEST WAY TO LENGTHEN OUT OUR DAYS IS TO WALK STEADILY AND WITH A PURPOSE." *Charles Dickens*

The objective of this book is to help you get the most out of your pedometer. It will try to inspire you, motivate you, help you to a healthier life and enable you to integrate exercise into your weight-loss programme. The pedometer has already proved to be a valuable weapon in the war against obesity and, used seriously (which doesn't mean we won't be having fun!), it can help you change your whole life.

Walking back to happiness

The popularity of the pedometer is not just a British phenomenon, it is a worldwide craze that has lasted so long because it works. If used correctly, noticeable improvements can be achieved over a period of just weeks. In next to no time, you will appreciate the everyday benefits:

- You won't be out of breath every time you climb the stairs.
- You'll discover muscle definition as your body tones up.
- Body fat will gradually disappear.
- Waist and hip sizes will diminish.
- You'll find ever new energy reserves.
- You'll feel less tired at the end of the day.
- Your brain will send out endorphins (feel-good chemicals) which means you'll feel happier!

Prevention really is the best form of cure

The use of a pedometer is recommended by, among others, the American Heart Association, the British Heart Foundation, the American Diabetes Association, Cancer Research, Diabetes UK and the British Medical Association. Their research has shown that a significant amount of walking on a daily basis can help to protect against a number of lifestyle-related diseases which include:

- Heart disease
- Cardiovascular disease
- High cholesterol
- High blood pressure
- Some cancers
- Strokes
- Osteoporosis
- Depression
- Stress

Talking the talk

The idea is simple: walking helps burn off the excess calories we consume. The more we walk, the more calories we will devour. If your aim is to maintain a healthy lifestyle, you will find ideas, tips and suggestions of ways to reach your step target and maintain that level. You will find the fill-in chart on pages 124–191 ideal for keeping your records. These will be of even more use for those aiming to lose weight as comments about diet and weight can also be written down.

Walking the walk

Studies around the world have reached a pretty unanimous conclusion that taking 10,000 steps is a reasonable daily target for the normal adult. That's about five miles, which probably sounds a lot to you. The average person in the western world takes about 4,000 steps a day, so somehow we have to find another 6,000 in between working, seeing to the kids, meeting friends and, well, living our lives. That's where this book will help you. It's amazing how easily you can find more steps – walking the kids to school, window shopping or even leaving the remote control for the television on top of the set .

One step at a time

The great thing about the pedometer is that you set your own goals and monitor your own progress. If you lead a pretty sedentary life and don't take much exercise, you'll probably find the idea of doubling your activity overnight pretty daunting. Don't worry. This book will help you set your own reachable targets, encourage you to stretch yourself a little more when you are ready and provide support when you are finding things too challenging.

Motivation

So, imagine you've had your new pedometer for a few days now. You have set yourself a target and, eagerly checking your steps at every possible opportunity, you find you are reaching it comfortably. You have discovered fabulous ways of clocking up steps – walking on the spot while washing up or walking the long way round to the shops – and are even sometimes exceeding your target.

Now imagine yourself in a week, a month or even three months' time. Has the novelty worn off? Does the washing up seem enough of a drag as it is without marching while you do it? Is that long route march to the shops making you miss exciting episodes of your favourite soap? If this programme is going to work, it will involve a fairly long-term commitment. That means starting the way you mean to continue and planning ahead. Below are a few ideas to bear in mind:

1. Prepare yourself properly with the correct clothing and attitudes.
2. Set targets that are achievable but not too easy.
3. Try to be creative in finding methods of clocking up steps.
4. Discover which motivation techniques work for you.
5. Monitor your progress regularly but not over-obsessively.
6. Plan a long-term change to your lifestyle.
7. Learn to enjoy walking for its own sake.

The chapters of this book will deal with all of these issues and provide sensible advice and techniques. If you manage to increase your daily step total even by a small amount over an extended period of time, you will feel the benefit. But try not to become despondent, expect the excitement of clocking up a handful of steps to wear off pretty quickly and look for fresh new ways to keep yourself motivated.

Did You Know
On average, every minute you spend walking can extend your life by 1.5–2 minutes!

Walking part of the way

Walking your 10,000 steps a day is going to set you on the road to a healthier body, but if you are really serious about staying fit, you will have to consider some other aspects of your lifestyle.

- Does your diet include a variety of foods?
- Are you sleeping well and regularly?
- Are you a smoker?
- Do you regularly consume alcoholic drinks?

As you will discover, it is possible to lose weight through a walking programme. You'll be burning off around 350 extra calories on a 10,000-step day, but those pounds will come off much quicker if you consider:

- Cutting down on fried, fatty and sweet foods
- Upping your intake of fruit and vegetables
- Being more careful about your portion sizes
- Being aware of the dangers of alcoholic or fizzy drinks and snacks

The forthcoming chapters will detail how simple changes in your lifestyle, in conjunction with a daily step plan, can lead to significant weight loss, a healthy body and the opportunity to lead a fuller and more enjoyable life.

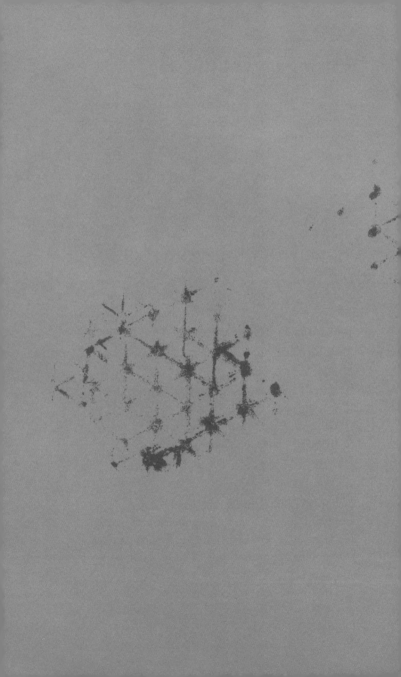

3 Using your Pedometer

"OF ALL EXERCISES, WALKING IS THE BEST." Thomas Jefferson

Do you think pedometers are a recent gadget, a gimmick that, perhaps like step routines, bullworkers and cycling machines will be here today and gone tomorrow? Well, think again. People have been counting steps ever since their Neanderthal ancestors left the jungle for that long walk across the savannah. Those unstoppable marchers, the Romans, defined a mile as 2,000 steps and the great genius Leonardo da Vinci came up with drawings for an accurate pedometer in the fifteenth century. Three hundred years later, the American President, Thomas Jefferson, bought one in France and introduced it to the New World.

Stepping back in time – the history of pedometers

Still not convinced? Fast-forward to Japan, 1965, where the first commercially produced pedometer was made available. As the 1964 Olympics in Tokyo inspired the Japanese to get healthy, Dr Yoshiro Hatano developed the "Manpo-kei" programme – literally translated it means "10,000 steps". When the public responded, the government introduced an industrial standard that any pedometer sold had to be accurate to within three per cent. Today, they are still using them. A recent survey found that, on average, each Japanese household owns three pedometers.

In the USA and the UK, fitness fanatics were the first to realize their potential but it was not long before medical experts saw this digital accessory as a weapon in the fight against obesity. Thousands began to walk for their health. Fast-food outlets and cereal manufacturers jumped on the "healthy" bandwagon, and stars like Robbie Williams, Caprice and Cameron Diaz were seen out checking their step tally. In the UK, explorer Sir Ranulph Fiennes became patron of the Move 4 Health campaign and, in parliament, fitness guru Joanna Hall led a group of MPs – including Health Secretary John Reid and Culture Secretary Tessa Jowell – on an awareness-raising programme.

Will it last? The UK's Countryside Agency, which launched a Walking For Health initiative in 2001, suggests it will. Half of a sample of people who began using pedometers two years ago are still using them. And 93 per cent say they are still walking more as a result. Today, estimates put the number of pedometers in use in the UK at around two million – and there are many more in use around the world!

> **TOP TIP**
> Keep a pair of walking shoes in your car, just in case an opportunity to walk arises.

How the pedometer works

There's no need for you to understand the finer scientific points, but just so you are assured that it's not magic, here's how your pedometer counts your steps.

1 A lever mechanism inside the pedometer moves up and down as you move (try shaking it; it will think you are walking – though this isn't an acceptable way of clocking up steps!).

2 With each firm movement of the lever, an electrical pulse is recorded. So, when your foot hits the ground, your pedometer will register one step.

3 The step is then automatically added to the tally on the screen, displaying your accumulated total.

4 When you press the reset button, the pedometer will return the counter to zero. You are therefore able to start the counter afresh each day.

Wearing your pedometer

If your pedometer is going to record every step, it is important that you wear it correctly and check its position regularly. As people come in different shapes and sizes, so finding the most accurate position is often a matter of trial and error. But remember that the pedometer must be secure and clipped at right angles to the ground. Follow these guidelines when fixing your pedometer to your clothes:

- Hold the pedometer so the display counter faces outwards.
- Slide the clip onto your belt or waistband halfway between your belly button and your hip.

- If you are right-footed, try and wear the pedometer on the right-hand side, while left-footers should move it to the left.
- Line the pedometer up with the centre of your knee-cap.
- Make sure it is vertical and directly in line with your foot.
- Wear it with pride! The pedometer will work better if it is not inhibited by clothes.

Alternative positions for your pedometer

For various reasons, you may not wish to wear the pedometer on your hip. Although research has shown this is the most effective position, there are some alternatives you can try.

- If you are wearing a dress without a waistband, try attaching the pedometer with a safety pin or clip it on to the waistband of your underwear.
- Try hanging the pedometer on a string – or lanyard – around your neck.
- It should be possible to receive an accurate reading, if you manage to clip it to a boot or shoe.

Note for those with more expansive tummies

If you have a protruding belly – don't worry we'll deal with that later! – you may need to find a position where the pedometer won't be pushed out of its vertical position. Try placing it on the side of the hip before resorting to the above options.

How not to wear your pedometer

- Don't put it in your pocket.
- Don't clip it to an angled pocket.
- Don't attach it near your belly button.
- Don't allow it to edge out of position as you walk.
- Don't let your belly push it from its vertical position.

Testing your pedometer

- Attach the pedometer as advised above.
- Take 20 steps.
- Stop and read the pedometer display.
- If it reads between 19 and 21, you have found an effective position.
- If it reads less or fails to register, move the pedometer towards your hip and try again.

Why the pedometer might not work

1 The most probable reason is that you are wearing it incorrectly. See page 36 for instructions on how to position it for maximum sensitivity.

2 Pedometers have been known to work even after a spin in the washing machine or a dunk in the toilet bowl. If something like that happens to your pedometer, remove the battery immediately (see point 3 below) and leave the pedometer in a warm dry place for at least 24 hours. Insert a new battery and cross your fingers…

3 If the reading becomes dim, it could be that the battery is running out – they generally last 1–2 years. Use a coin to open the battery compartment and carefully remove the old battery so as not to break the silver flap underneath. You should be able to buy a replacement from most normal electrical stores. This should be fitted, making sure the + end is facing upwards.

DID YOU KNOW?

The average person in the UK or the USA only walks 4,500 steps a day.

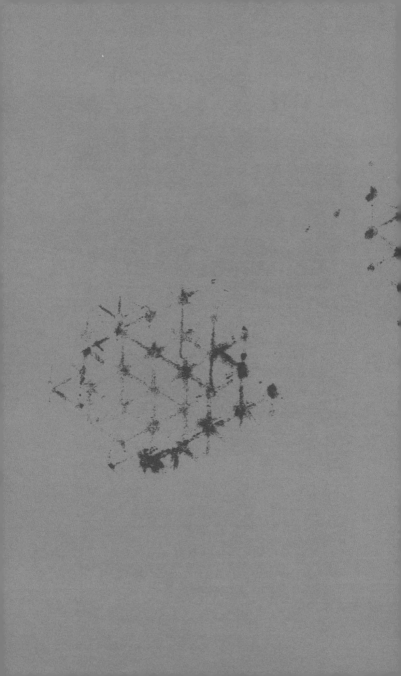

4 Best Foot Forward

Proceed with caution

If you have any doubts or concerns about your ability to perform a moderate amount of exercise, now is the time to see your doctor or medical adviser. You should not attempt to undertake vigorous or taxing physical activity without gradually developing and maintaining an appropriate level of fitness. This is particularly important for anyone aged 30 or over.

Equipment

You are, of course, already in possession of one of the most important pieces of equipment – the pedometer. What else you require is largely down to personal preference, but you will probably find that, as you become more immersed in a walking programme, you will wish to be better equipped. Alternatively, buying specific kit may be your way of motivating yourself, in which case go ahead and "flash the plastic".

Shoes

There is, however, one overriding requirement: an appropriate pair of shoes. Your everyday work or casual shoes will obviously suffice for the kind of activities you already perform, but you should have some pre-selected footwear for your longer outings. It is your choice whether you opt for trainers, running shoes, walking boots or even a scuffed-up pair of Kickers, but bear in mind the following considerations:

- Ensure the footwear has been worn in and will not leave you with blisters and corns.
- The shoes or trainers should support the heel firmly and leave enough room for you to wiggle your toes.
- Try to find a pair with a flexible, cushioned sole that will absorb some of the shock of your step.
- Are they suitable for all the kinds of weather you are likely to encounter? Will they be waterproof in a snap storm and are they made of a breathable material (preferably leather) that won't leave you feeling that they are two sizes two small in a sunny spell?
- Check they are going to last you a reasonable time – you don't want to have to break in a new pair just as your programme gets tougher.
- They may be comfortable enough for a quick stroll through the park, but how will they feel after a bracing 50-minute walk?

Cold weather clothing

You might be out for some time so consider what you wear carefully. Although you might feel the cold at first, you will warm up after a short while and need to remain comfortable.

Remember:

- To wear layers of clothing which trap heat but can be removed as you warm up.
- To keep each layer as lightweight as possible; you don't want to be lugging a heavy overcoat around.

- To wear a hat – over 30 per cent of body heat is lost through the head.
- If you feel the cold, consider wearing thermal underwear, gloves, and a thick, or extra, pair of socks, although avoid woollens (especially scarves) that may cause you to perspire too much. Those with poor circulation may also appreciate the small, portable handwarmers that are now widely available.

Warm weather clothing

When the sun is shining, the main consideration is that you consume plenty of water (see page 114). However, also bear the following in mind:

- Dress lightly. You may not think you look good in T-shirt and shorts but it's better than completing your walk, red-faced and clad in sweat-drenched clothes.
- Remember the sun can easily harm your skin – wear a high-factor suncream (SPF30 or above) on all exposed body parts and even sunblock on your face and ears.
- A lightweight hat or cap will protect your head from the worst of the sun's rays.
- Other optional extras include sunglasses, towelling wristbands and headbands and refreshing wipes.

Rainwear

At some point during your walking programme you are going to get caught in a surprise downpour – guaranteed. It's just a calculation of time spent outdoors and the frequency of rain showers. So...

- Like a good cub scout, be prepared. Check the forecasts.
- Find a showerproof hat you are comfortable with. If possible avoid using an umbrella as it will inhibit your movement.
- Wear a coat with a hood or, better still, invest in a cheap foldaway plastic raincoat. However unfashionable, they are lightweight – useful both when carrying and when wearing them while working up a brisk pace – and they will keep you pretty dry.
- If you are intending to head out for several long walks, it may also be worthwhile buying a pair of lightweight showerproof trousers. There's nothing like being wet through for ruining a good walk.

How to walk properly

You've been doing it ever since you were very small. Surely no one needs to be told how to put one foot in front of another? True enough, but you want to cover the ground as quickly, smoothly and with as little jarring to your bones as possible, so it is worth taking note of how you stand, step and move. "Serious" walking will also use more calories and help tone your muscles – and you just might find you're not arriving late for anything any more! However, please don't let this put you off – if you feel it is all too much to remember, work on one thing at a time or intersperse periods of "serious" walking with a relaxing dawdle or saunter.

Posture

- Stand as tall and straight as possible – think of how a soldier marches. Not only will this be good for your back, but your whole body will benefit so much more than if you shuffle along, hunched up and crooked.
- Keep your head upright. It's pretty heavy and, if you let it hang, it will put strain on your neck and back. Generally try to look ahead about five or six yards (4.5–5.5 m) – as if you were looking across a road – but still keep an eye out for those uneven pavements or potholes!
- Draw in your stomach – you'll find your chest is immediately raised (and, perhaps, there's a little more room around your waistband).
- Clench those buttocks – this time your back will follow, straightening up and losing its arch.

Arms

- Swinging your arms properly can give you extra momentum to make your walk easier and use up more calories – turning a walk into a workout.

- Bend your arms at the elbow so the upper and lower parts are at right angles. Your swing should now be quicker and more controlled.
- Keep your fingers together but relaxed – don't clench your fists or you'll find the rest of your body tensing up as well.
- Swing your left arm forwards as your right foot moves forward and your right arm moves in time with your left foot.
- Keep your arms straight. Your elbows should tuck in beside your ribs and your hands should not venture past the centre of the body.
- There is no need to swing wildly. A short, controlled, regular movement is enough to aid a brisk stroll.

Step

- Be aware of how your feet make contact with the ground. Feel how you actually walk with your heel, the ball of your foot and the toes.
- Aim for smoothness, avoiding jerky or jarring steps.
- Push one foot forwards from the toe. Let the other leg remain relaxed.
- Let your heel hit the ground first and roll the step through to the toe.
- Push off with the other leg. Don't bounce or slap your feet down, just keep the movement consistent and relaxed.

Stride

- Find a length of stride – as short as possible – that you are comfortable with.
- Your stride should see your leg extending further behind your body than in front. The push-off is where your power will come from.
- Stick to it. As long as you are comfortable you should always set out with the same length stride.

If you want to increase speed, increase the rate of your steps. Don't be tempted to lengthen it in order to go faster as this could easily lead to muscle injury.

Five things to remember

1 Overstriding – your steps are too long and you're bouncing along. Your heels, knees and shins will tell you it's a no-no.
2 Arms – flapping? Hanging? Chicken-winging? Bend those elbows for maximum results.
3 Water – a loss of two per cent of body fluids causes a 20 per cent reduction in performance in both physical and mental activities.
4 Clothes – wear less rather than overdress. If you get cold, up the pace.
5 Cut your toenails – doing so will help you avoid bruised nails, athlete's foot and cuts to your toes… look after your feet, you're going to need them!

Walking uphill

Walking uphill is more demanding than walking on the level: walking up a 15 per cent (1 in 7) slope uses over 30 per cent more calories than walking on the level. However, it will put stress on your calves and the front of your thighs as well as possibly leaving you a little breathless. Do:

1 Warm up before tackling a steep hill. Spend a few minutes walking on the flat beforehand or do some of the stretching exercises on page 75.
2 Keep your feet as flat as possible with heels down; don't walk on you toes.
3 Let the thigh lift and pull the knee through. The thighs are the strongest muscles in the body, while the calves should only help keep the lower leg operating smoothly.
4 Take care not to overstep. The knee should not be raised more than six inches.
5 Shorten your stride, but increase or keep your pace at the same level.
6 Lean forward slightly, but keep your balance.
7 Keep a steady rhythm going. If it helps, sing a song or chant a mantra as you go.
8 Stop if your breathing becomes too deep. You should be able to hold a normal conversation without taking gasps in between words.

Walking downhill

Of course, walking downhill is much easier, but surprisingly it can still be a valuable exercise. Although it takes about the same amount of energy as walking on the level, walking down a steep hill will increase your exertion – and research by the American Heart Association has proved it can be beneficial in decreasing blood sugar levels. Here you need to watch out that your muscles don't work too hard to maintain balance and you need to be careful about the impact on certain joints, especially the ankles and the knees. Try to:

- Lean back a little to keep your back straight.
- Dig your heels in gently to take some of the strain off your knee, and on steeper slopes keep your knees slightly bent.
- Maintain a normal or even slightly shortened stride. Consider using small quick steps so your weight is transferred between your feet before the full impact of the step is felt.
- Keep your balance – if necessary choose a zigzagging path down the hill.
- Don't go too fast.

Walking faster

As you become more confident, you may wish to try and gain more from your walk by increasing your speed. Here, you should not alter your technique too much but concentrate on:

1 Standing tall and keeping your eyes on the horizon
2 Taking quicker, but not longer steps. As you walk, every now and then, count how many steps you take in a minute and try to do a couple more each time.
3 Remembering to bend your arms – use short, quick swings that get your feet moving faster.
4 Pushing off from your toes. With each step, imagine you are showing someone behind you the sole of your shoe.

Among walkers, you may find "brisk walking" defined as 15 minutes per mile, but for most beginners this is too fast. If you're just starting to walk seriously, do what seems brisk to you and gradually try to increase your pace. Try interval training (see page 112) where you aim to walk fast for short periods, returning to a normal pace in between.

TOP TIP
Take up pitch and putt or even golf.

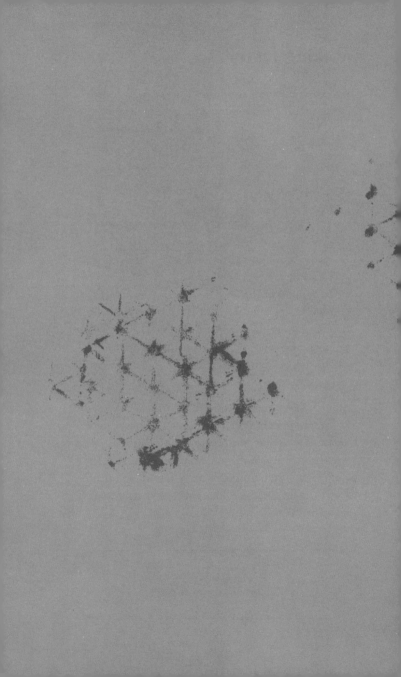

5 How Fit Are You?

"FITNESS — IF IT CAME IN A BOTTLE, EVERYBODY WOULD HAVE A GREAT BODY." Cher

To begin setting our objectives for getting fitter
we need to have some idea of our starting point.
If you are a fairly sedentary (i.e. don't generally walk
very much), perhaps overweight, person, your realistic
goals are going to be different from those of a young,
fit man or woman. Once again, however, it is essential
that, if you have any doubts about your ability to
undertake serious exercise or feel it could cause health
problems, you should consult your GP or health
expert before starting on this, or any other,
diet or fitness programme.

Assess your health

Answer these questions as honestly as possible and tot
up your score giving one point for answering (a); two
points for answering (b); three for (c) and four for (d).
Then look at the results as a guide to setting your
personal objectives.

1 **How old are you?**
   a) Over 50
   b) 40–50
   c) 30–40
   d) 16–30

2 **Would you consider yourself...** (see the Body
   Mass Index chart on page 57 if you are unsure)
   a) Obese
   b) Overweight
   c) Underweight
   d) A normal weight for your height?

3 Do you take part in any sports, exercise classes or any other regular physically demanding activities (such as an hour's gardening)?
   a) Never
   b) Every now and then
   c) About once a week
   d) Daily

4 How often do you take a five-minute (or longer) walk in one day?
   a) Never
   b) Once or twice
   c) Three or four times
   d) More than four times

5 How often do you take a 20-minute (or longer) walk?
   a) Never or rarely
   b) Once a week
   c) Once every few days
   d) Every day

6 If you walk quickly up an average flight of steps (around 15) in a house, are you:
   a) Gasping for breath?
   b) Breathing heavily but able to talk?
   c) Back to normal in ten seconds or so?
   d) Breathing relatively normally?

Results

6–10 Try out your pedometer on a normal day. You are probably walking 2–3,000 steps a day. You should be looking for gradual progress, moving on to the next stage when you are ready. It is important that you don't rush to the 10,000-step goal. If you are constantly struggling to meet your targets, reassess your daily goals. This isn't a race and you will get there in good time if you persist.

10–12 Although you are probably not walking a great deal at the moment, you should be capable of increasing your step count reasonably quickly. If you take things steadily – adding 750 or so steps to your target each week – you should reach the 10,000-step mark by the latter part of the programme.

11–17 As a reasonably fit person you should be able to build up to 10,000 steps quite quickly. Your problems might come in finding the necessary motivation. Remember to keep setting yourself new targets – try increasing your pace until you are beginning to feel breathless or increasing your target number of steps to 12,000.

18–24 Your general fitness level should enable you to manage the daily 10,000-step target pretty easily from the start. Once you are sure you are comfortable with this, start pushing yourself to more difficult objectives. Try some walks against the clock, setting yourself a time limit, or why not decide to join the superfit and go for the 20,000?

Did You Know?
Thirty-seven per cent of coronary heart disease deaths are related to inactivity, compared to 19 per cent related to smoking.

Measuring your progress

As you continue with your programme, you will hopefully begin to notice improvements in your fitness and weight. But if you wish to chart your improvements, here are some suggested methods.

Scales

As a quick check, getting on the bathroom scales (that's one more step!) is a fair means of assessing your progress. But remember that your weight fluctuates during the month and you could be recording fluid rather than fat loss.

Body mass index (BMI)

In recent years, body mass index (BMI) has become the medical standard used to determine whether patients are underweight, normal, overweight or obese. To find your BMI, divide your weight in kilos (1 lb = 0.45 kg) by your height in metres (1 ft = 30.48 cm) squared. For example, if your height is 180 cm (6 ft) and your weight is 75 kilos (165 lbs), your BMI is 23.1.

Alternatively, you could enter the details of your weight and size on one of the many internet sites such as www.bbc.co.uk/health/healthy_living/your_weight/bmiimperial_index.shtml

For a rough check, you can consult the graph below.

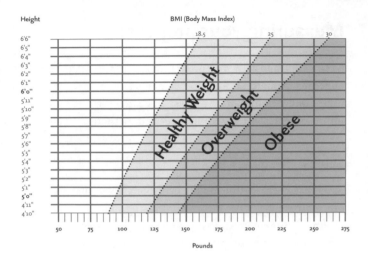

This measurement provides a useful gauge, but bear in mind if you are muscular or athletic – and maybe you soon will be! – that it will overestimate your BMI.

Body-fat percentage

Remember, weight loss doesn't always mean fat loss. As you exercise regularly, your body will have more lean muscle mass and less fat. This can be charted through body-fat percentage tests, which simply determine the percentage of fat your body contains. They are available at gyms and some of the well-known chemists, or if you can take a number of measurements yourself and enter them on a web site. There are a number of sites which will calculate it for you including www.weightlossforgood.co.uk/body_fat_calculator.htm Once you have your result, consult the chart to assess your body-fat level.

Classification	Women (% fat)	Men (% fat)
Essential fat	10–12	2–4
Athletes	14–20	6–13
Fitness	21–24	14–17
Acceptable	25–31	18–25
Obese	32 plus	25 plus

Heart beat

The rate at which your heart is beating is a great indicator of your general level of fitness. Your heart will beat at different rates depending on your activity. The rate will be at its lowest when you are sleeping and resting, and higher when you are exercising (or attending a job interview or even while watching a cliff-hanging episode of a soap opera). It is useful, therefore, to be able to measure your "resting" heart beat, what level it reaches when you exercise rigorously and how quickly it returns to normal. But first you need to ascertain how to take your pulse (heart rate) easily.

Some people find taking their pulse very easy, while others need some practice. The first place to try is your wrist. If you are right-handed, place the pads of your index and middle fingers on the underside of your left wrist – about an inch below the thumb base. Press down lightly – if you feel a regular "throbbing", you've found it. If the pulse is too faint or you can't feel anything, try taking your pulse on the side of your neck. Lifting your chin very slightly and, again with the sensitive pads of your index and middle fingers, feel just by the centre of your throat until you detect a pulsing sensation.

Once you're sure you have found your pulse, look at a clock with a second hand or a watch and, beginning at 0, count the number of beats for a period of 10 seconds. Multiply the final number of beats by six and you will have determined your "heartbeats per minute".

Resting heart rate

As you get fitter, your resting heart rate should decrease. As the heart becomes more efficient at pumping blood around the body, it needs fewer beats to pump the same amount.

Take your resting heart rate (the number of beats per minute) a few minutes (2–5) after you wake up in the morning and while you are still in bed. Give your body some time to adjust to the change from sleeping before taking your pulse.

The heart beats about 60–90 times a minute (the average resting heart rate for a woman is 75 beats per minute and 70 for a man). As you become fitter, you should see your resting heart rate come down.

Recovery heart rate

Another good guide for those aiming at a high fitness level is to take your pulse a minute after exercising. By this time your pulse should be returning to its normal rate. As you get fitter, it should return much more rapidly.

Rockport Walking Test

The scientifically (and therefore fairly difficult to calculate) accepted Rockport Walking Test provides a much more accurate means of tracking your fitness. It is done by measuring your aerobic power (VO2max). This test requires you to warm up for five or more minutes until you feel ready. You should then walk as fast as possible for one mile (approx. 2,000 steps), timing how long you take to complete it. When you have finished, take your pulse rate immediately and write it down. When you've recovered and are back home with a glass of water, apply the following calculation:

139.168 - (0.388 x age in years) - (0.077 x weight in lbs) - (3.265 x walk time in minutes) - (0.156 x heart rate in beats per minute).

Note: men should add 6.318 to their total.

Again, if you find the maths a little daunting, there are a number of sites on the internet that will calculate it for you. One such is www.brianmac.demon.co.uk/rockport.htm

---

TOP TIP

Going shopping? Take a lap or two around the shopping centre before going into stores.

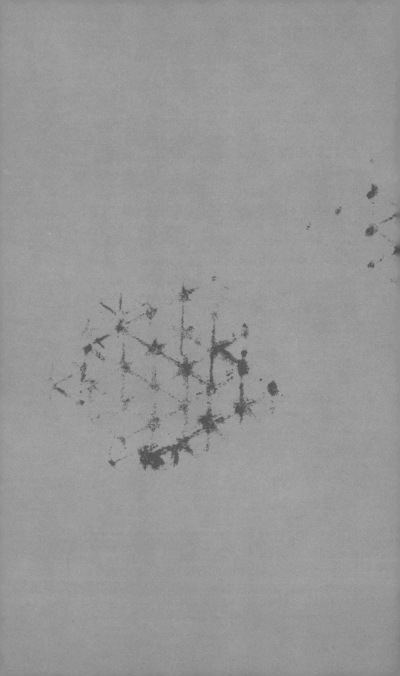

6 First Steps

"THE DISTANCE IS NOTHING; IT IS ONLY
THE FIRST STEP THAT IS DIFFICULT."
Madame du Deffand

"I can't because…"

For every reason – fitness, weight, happiness – we can come up with for getting out and getting healthy, it's a sure bet that we could come up with twice as many reasons to stay on the sofa eating things that aren't good for us: "My knee feels a funny… "; "I haven't got the right shoes… "; "There's something good on TV… "; "I have to eat what the kids eat… ". You know them all, so let's dismiss the top ten, so you can get them out of the way and get walking…

1 I can't see the point in starting
If you are too overweight, too unfit and have too unhealthy a lifestyle even to begin walking, just forget about the results for now and simply walk when you can. Set yourself some easily achievable targets, focusing on your next goal. You'll be amazed at how soon the benefits become apparent.

2 I haven't got the time
You will have to work a little at this, but millions of others succeed, so why can't you? As you will discover, it is possible to fit work, kids, housework, friends and fun around a daily 10,000-step target. It's time to get organized.

3 I'm not the sporty type
No one is asking you to do an intense workout – getting sweaty, red-faced and gasping for air. And you don't need to squeeze into a leotard or fluorescent leggings. The great thing is that this is something you do every

day. All you need is to do it a little more – and if you do need one, you can shower in the privacy of your own home.

4 I haven't got the energy

If you can, just force yourself outside; you'll find that your get-up-and-go hasn't got up and gone but is waiting for you to kick-start it. Light exercise will leave you feeling more invigorated than before and, as you become fitter and eat more healthily, it will become easier and easier to keep moving.

5 There's nowhere around here to walk

Walking doesn't just have to be up hill and down dale. It can be part of your normal day, a shopping excursion or an exploration of a housing estate.
You'll be amazed at what you can discover about your local area or your own thoughts on a short stroll.

6 Everyone thinks I'll fail

Who needs a better motivation than being able to prove the doubters wrong. There is only one person who needs to believe you can reach your goals – YOU.
If you think your friend, or partner, or parent will support you, then enlist their help. If not, just don't tell them – and enjoy their reaction even more when you succeed.

7 I've no one to walk with

Of course it's fun walking with a friend or even a walking partner and, if you are desperate for company, there are walking clubs you can join (see page 118). But even if you are lucky enough to have a companion,

you'll still find yourself walking alone sometimes.
And you'll get to enjoy it. This is when you can be alone
with your thoughts and when you can push yourself to
your goals without considering whether you are too fast
or slow for your partner.

8   Diets never work for me – I'm naturally overweight

First of all, this is not a diet. This is a way of leading a
healthy lifestyle which, if you are overweight, should
lead to you losing weight. A tiny, tiny percentage of the
population is genetically obese. That probably doesn't
mean you. It's time to check what you're eating and lace
up those shoes…

9   I'm not quite ready

If you are a "never do today what you can put off until
tomorrow" person, you'll find an endless supply of
excuses – "It's too cold"; "I'll wait for a nice day"; "I'm
feeling a bit stressed at the moment"; "I'll wait until the
first of the month" – but this isn't some kind of ordeal
you are going to put yourself through. It can begin with
a short walk around the block. Forget your petty
distractions, the time to start is always NOW.

10 The pedometer is not working

When all else fails, blame the equipment. If your
pedometer does not appear to be counting your steps
properly, return to page 36 and make sure you have
positioned it correctly. If you've counted 30 steps and
it is only registering 28, don't worry. You are not in a
competition with anyone except yourself and, as long as
you use the same pedometer, your progress will be
deadly accurate.

Ten thousand steps into one day won't go?

Twenty-first century life is so varied that it is difficult to prescribe a timetable to ensure everybody has an opportunity to walk at least 10,000 steps. Shift workers, part-time workers, working parents, pensioners – all will have different lifestyles to work round. Working on the basis that you are already walking around 3–5,000 steps a day, you will be looking for roughly another hour's walking time. You could choose to do this in one walk, but, equally, if you are on a busy schedule, you could break it down into as many bite-sized strolls as you want. It is also worth remembering that you can carry steps over to the next day, but make sure you don't go too far overdrawn.

Nine-to-fivers

Many people have found it relatively easy to fit their steps into a normal working day. Getting to and from work provides an obvious opportunity, but walking to talk to, or leave a message for, a colleague instead of emailing or phoning them can also increase your tally by a surprising amount. Lunchtimes also provide a valuable opportunity for a bit of window shopping or a muscle-stretching stroll. It is amazing how much better it can make you feel in the afternoon as well.

Potterers

You could be unemployed, a pensioner or a homemaker, but your day is still made up of a number of elements, which may include chores, trips to the shops, or the library, or meeting friends. Your task is to think about these elements and try to work out how you could fit in your extra steps or perhaps schedule your day to allow for a reasonably serious walk in the evening. Your time is sure to be as valuable as everyone else's, but when you start to think of how many steps you can fit around your activities you, too, will be surprised.

Did You Know?

The average person takes 9,000 steps each day. In a lifetime, that is 3.5 trips around the Earth.

Social whirl

If you are one of those people who live life on the hoof – flitting from one engagement to another – there is a plus and a minus. The plus is that your social whirl is probably providing an above average number of steps already. The minus? You are going to have to work hard and make some social sacrifices to make up the balance. Consider meeting friends 20 minutes later than usual (sometimes you may wait that long for them to arrive anyway!) and walk some of the way, or – even better – invite them to come on a stroll with you and let them catch the walking bug as well.

Working parents

Congratulations! Or should that be commiserations? You are part of the group that will find it toughest to produce those extra steps. But, if you've read this far, you should already have the motivation. Hopefully, you'll find further inspiration in the following chapters, but consider how much of your time is taken up ferrying the kids to and from school, out to friends' houses, or football training, or to the cinema. Are any of these walkable? And what about your partner – is it time he or she spent more quality time with the children and helped you become a more contented, healthier person?

One step at a time

This is your programme – planned by you, measured by you and judged by you. The only person to suffer if you cheat is yourself. But… this is a long-term, perhaps a lifetime, programme and it is essential to stick at it. Research has proved that people who can stick with a new pattern of behaviour for six months usually make it a habit. That six-month mark should be one of your primary objectives. In order to make that you will need to:

- Persevere – if it was easy, we'd be doing it already.
- Enjoy – be one of the converts who discover a real joy in walking.
- Fail – allow yourself to fail. It's only by getting back on again that you learn to succeed.
- Relax – don't push yourself so far that it becomes impossible.
- Reward – allow yourself treats and days off if it helps keep you going. But not too many!

Walk/don't walk

Unless you have a fair amount of free time in your day, it is advisable to plan where you will be collecting your steps. Think what your plans are for that day, or even for the next two or three days.

- Try to find at least 20 minutes or half an hour when you can do some serious walking.
- Identify those opportunities when you can find an extra five or ten minutes' walking time.
- Decide on your strategy: are you going to create time to walk or fit it in around your daily activities.
- You might decide you will do as much as you can during the day and "top up" your steps in the evening. If you do, ensure that you don't have conflicting engagements.

Think about where you are going to walk. Busy roads, muddy lanes, crowded pavements and rugged fields can all make walking a much more unpleasant experience.

TOP TIP

The first four to five weeks are the most critical period in keeping to a physical routine. Keep your walking programme going for at least a month to give yourself a fair chance.

Safety

Walking is one of the safest forms of exercise you can undertake. You are able to look around you at all times and you progress at a speed where you are able to stop quickly. However, there are still certain precautions you should take and dangers of which you should remain aware.

- If possible let someone know where you are heading.
- Try to carry a mobile phone – and make sure it is charged!
- Carry some form of identification – a driving licence, company ID etc.
- If you have one, carry your organ/tissue donor card.
- Have your wits about you. Don't go out if you feel sleepy or drowsy.

Trucks and cars present the greatest threat to pedestrians. Make sure you are aware of any traffic around you and:

- Where possible, stick to pavements, sidewalks and footpaths.
- If there is no footpath, walk on the side of the road so you can see oncoming traffic.
- In the daytime, wear white or brightly coloured clothing. At night, wear something reflective.
- Take care at crossroads and use pedestrian crossings correctly.
- If you decide to wear iPod or Walkman headphones, keep them at a level where you can hear oncoming traffic.

Keep looking around you. There are many other pitfalls for the unwary walker. Some are merely irritating, but others could result in injury:

- Dogs – keep a safe distance from all dogs, particularly those not on a leash. If an unleashed dog approaches you, walk calmly on. Don't run or try to intimidate the animal.
- Uneven pavements – keep an eye out for uneven pavements if you are walking briskly. A trip could result in a nasty bruise or sprain.
- Lamposts and bollards – try not to get too distracted so that you don't see what you are walking into (it happens!). In particular, keep an eye out for midriff-height bollards, they can be very painful!
- Cyclists: more and more cyclists seem to have taken – usually illegally – to our pavements. Don't get angry and try to knock them off. Step aside if necessary and, if you are still enraged when you get home, pen a letter to your local paper.
- People – be aware of who is around you. If you see a suspicious group or person, cross the street or turn round and head for a safe area – a busy street or a house that you are familiar with. The chances of you getting into any trouble are very slight, but always do what your instincts tell you, and you'll be clocking up more steps in the process.

Night walking

Walking after dark carries its own safety concerns and yet the tranquility and atmosphere of the evening (or early morning) can make it an even better experience than walking in the day. If you have concerns about night walking, you might consider joining a gym where you can use a treadmill. But if you are venturing out, here are a few tips to make you feel more secure when night walking:

- Whenever possible, go with a friend or a walking group.
- Stick to populated streets or late-opening shopping centres and malls and avoid areas you know to be trouble spots, such as teenage hangouts, notorious estates, or roads full of pubs and clubs.
- Carry a torch if you have to walk along roads without street lighting.
- Wear reflective clothing – belts, jackets or tabards – and flashing red lights which are available from all cycling shops.
- Have a route in mind. Know exactly where you are going and show this by walking confidently and alertly with your head up.
- Carry a portable alarm for use in an emergency. If you feel you have to carry a weapon, make sure it is legal to do so and that you have been trained to use it properly.
- Do walk with a dog, if you have one. Even the smallest dog can deter a would-be assailant.

Warming-up

You may think this is time that could be better spent walking, but an effective warming-up and warming-down session can save you a thousand aches and pains and could even prevent serious muscular injury. It just involves a few stretching exercises to flex the muscles you will use on your walk and you'll find the more often you do the stretches, the easier they will become.

As you begin to walk seriously, the repetitive movement of the muscles will tighten them and cause a lack of flexibility if it is not counterbalanced by another activity. Stretching is the means to ensure your muscles maintain the extra "play" they need. Obviously, the intensity of any warm-up will vary with the rigour of the exercise, but as you will eventually want to put some effort into your steps, here is a simple guide:

5–20 minutes at normal pace
For the first minute or so walk slightly slower than usual, then continue to ensure you are not overstriding and your pace is consistent.

5–20 minutes at an increased pace
Some basic stretching will help your long-term flexibility. When you start your walk, take it easy for a couple of minutes, increasing the pace every minute until you reach a peak at around the three-quarter mark. Then begin to decrease the pace again.

Over 20 minutes at normal pace

Spend a few minutes stretching. You will feel the benefit towards the end of your walk. When you reach the last few minutes of your walk, slow down and relax, allowing yourself to regain your normal breathing and pulse rate by the time you have finished. Then run through some basic warm-down stretches.

Over 20 minutes at an increased pace

Make sure you do a pretty full stretching session before setting out and even then take it easy for a few minutes. Once again, allow yourself a reasonable time at the end of the walk to help your body return to feeling normal and then spend five minutes warming down.

Stretching

Find a place where you can stretch without being disturbed and use a cushion if you find sitting down uncomfortable. Your stretches should be gradual so that you feel the muscle pull, but stop before it becomes uncomfortable. You will not benefit – and you can do yourself harm – by overstretching. When you begin to feel resistance from the muscle, stop and hold the position for 30 seconds or so. Do not "bounce", or try to force the muscle to stretch further.

TOP TIP

Go for a walk while waiting for a table at a restaurant.

Quadriceps stretch

1 Stand on your right leg, while steadying yourself with your right hand perhaps against a wall, or holding on to a piece of furniture.
2 Reach behind you with your left hand and grasp your left foot just above your toes.
3 Pull the foot directly back (not to one side or the other), so that the left heel touches the left buttock – or as close as you can comfortably get it. You will feel the stretch in the muscle at the front of the thigh.
4 Hold the position for up to 30 seconds and then release, slowly returning the foot to the ground.
5 Repeat the exercise while standing on your left leg to stretch the quadriceps muscle of the right leg.

Hamstring stretch

• Sit on the floor with one leg extended and the other bent out to the side with the foot against the inside of the extended leg's knee.
• Slowly lean forwards, keeping your lower back locked.
• Feel the stretch in the muscle at the back of your thigh.
• Hold the position for up to 20 seconds.
• Gently straighten your body.
• Repeat the exercise with the other leg.

Calf stretch

- Stand about a yard (1 metre) in front of a vertical surface – a wall, a door or, if you are outside, a tree.
- Lean forwards with your hands against the surface.
- Extend one leg forwards with the foot flat on the ground and keep the other foot flat on the floor.
- Keeping your back straight, push your back leg into the ground.
- Feel the stretch in the lower calf.
- Hold the position for up to 30 seconds.
- Gradually relax by transferring your weight to the other leg.
- Repeat the exercise using the other leg.

Ankle strengthening

- Sit with both feet on the floor.
- Straighten one leg without locking the knee.
- Lift it just off the floor.
- Draw 10 clockwise circles with your foot, moving only your ankles.
- Draw 10 anti-clockwise circles.
- Repeat the exercise using the other foot.

DID YOU KNOW?

People who walk 20–25 miles per week outlive people who don't walk by several years.

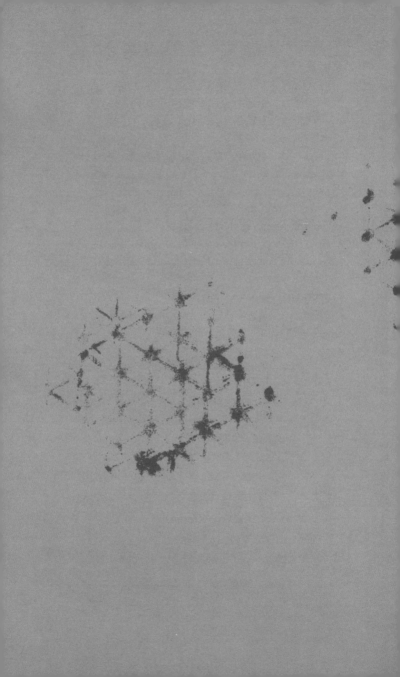

7 On the Road

"THE BODY OF MAN IS A MACHINE WHICH
WINDS ITS OWN SPRINGS."

J O De La Mettrie

At last, you're out and clocking up those steps. How does it feel? You are probably conscious of your pedometer and keen to check on your step tally. Have a look when you get to a convenient stop – check it is working and work out roughly how long it has taken you. The more you walk, the less you will notice it. You'll even be able to have a pretty good guess at how many steps you have done.

How fast?

What kind of pace are you walking at? Bear in mind the distance you have set out to walk; you don't want to be flagging when you have barely passed the halfway mark. If you are a beginner, start with some pretty short walks – of just 10 or 15 minutes' duration. Remember to keep pushing yourself, but don't forget that you should have enough puff to be able to carry on a conversation. If you are on your own, try talking to yourself silently. If you want to compare your pace, here is a very rough guide (as a more accurate result will also depend on hills, the weather conditions and the length of your stride etc) to how many steps you may have covered in 15 minutes:

Beginner	800
Average	1,500
Brisk	1,800
Fast	2,200

How far?

Of course, you are soon going to be curious – and some will get obsessive – about the distance you have covered. The total will depend on how much ground you are covering with each step, that is your stride length.

To gauge your stride length accurately, simply measure off a distance of 20 feet/240 inches (6 m/600 cm). Then count how many strides it takes to cover that distance and divide 240 (or 600) by that number. For example, if it took you 12 strides to cover 20 feet, your stride length would be 20 inches (or 50 cm). Here's a list of other typical stride lengths, based on the number of steps you might take to walk 20 feet:

10 steps	24-inch (60-cm) stride
11 steps	22-inch (57.5-cm) stride
12 steps	20-inch (50-cm) stride
13 steps	18½-inch (46.5 cm) stride
14 steps	17-inch (42-cm) stride
15 steps	16-inch (40-cm) stride

TOP TIP

When at the launderette, take a walk while your clothes are washing and again when they are in the dryer.

How many steps in a mile?

Step Length in Inches	Steps In One Mile
15	4,224
16	3,960
17	3,727
18	3,520
19	3,335
20	3,168
21	3,017
22	2,880
23	2,755
24	2,640
25	2,534
26	2,437
27	2,347
28	2,263
29	2,185
30	2,112
31	2,044
32	1,980
33	1,920
34	1,864
35	1,810
36	1,760

To convert your steps to miles see the chart at the end of the chapter.

Where does it hurt?

As a beginner, if you are pushing yourself even a little, you will almost inevitably feel some physical effects.

You should begin to feel the fabulous sensation of being physically tired. Unlike the spirit-sapping tiredness you feel after a bad day at work or an afternoon with a tantrum-turning toddler, your mind will still be alert and invigorated but your body will be crying out for a rest or a long soak in the bath. This is when you know you have worked as hard as you can and can justifiably expect to see some results.

There will also be times when, even hours after getting out of the bath, you continue to feel mild aches and pains. Don't panic or give up; there are many reasons why you may be feeling discomfort and most shouldn't involve hanging up your new trainers for good.

When you begin exercising, you are putting your body into a number of new situations which can be stressful. It won't always like it at first and these aches are its way of telling you so. But usually your body will get used to these changes pretty quickly and will recover in a surprisingly short space of time to emerge stronger. You will soon learn to understand the messages your body is sending, but the basic rules are:

1. If you are only in a little discomfort, soldier on, remembering to stick to your walking technique.
2. If the ache becomes more severe, stop as soon as you can.
3. If the pain prevents you from walking properly, rest immediately.
4. If the pain continues or becomes excruciating, see a medical expert.

Avoiding injuries – 10 tips

1 Warm up effectively.
2 Make sure footwear fits comfortably.
3 Concentrate on maintaining a correct stride length and technique.
4 Start out at a slow pace and slowly get faster.
5 Don't increase your steps by any more than 10 per cent each week.
6 Avoid dehydration – carry a bottle of water on long walks.
7 Choose your terrain – soft grass, dirt lanes, athletic tracks and treadmills are better than pavements.
8 Carry one or two plasters in case of blisters.
9 Slow down as you approach the final few minutes and warm down.
10 Have a long soak in the bath.

Shins

Aching shins are a very common complaint for beginners and walkers increasing their speed or distance. Shin splints are caused by putting too much stress on the muscles, which occurs through exercising too much, using an incorrect technique or by walking on hard terrain. They should get better as you progress.

Ankles

For overweight and novice walkers, weak ankles can be a serious problem. Work on the ankle-strengthening exercise on page 77 and avoid uneven terrain and rough country. Take care when stepping off pavements or turning sharply. If you twist an ankle, rest until you feel it strengthen and consider wearing an athletic support when walking.

Knees

Striking the foot down jarringly and going downhill too fast are major causes of knee injury. Most aches will disappear overnight but taking ibuprofen (always follow manufacturers' advice!) can temporarily numb the pain.

Heels

You should be walking with a low heel and you will benefit by generally wearing flat shoes until your feet have strengthened. Your heel may also be put under stress if you are hitting the ground with too flat a foot and you are rolling your foot inwards.

DID YOU KNOW?

The ancient Egyptians prescribed walking through a garden as a cure for the mad.

Blisters

Blisters develop where shoes and socks rub against the skin. Make sure that your shoes fit well and that your feet are dry. If a blister is already developing, or you feel that an area of your foot is likely to develop one, cover it with a blister pad before setting out.

Chafing

Where your clothes are wet through with sweat or rain, excessive rubbing can cause soreness. Areas that are particularly vulnerable are nipples, inner thighs and ribs. Take preventative action where possible: use petroleum jelly to lubricate some of these areas, wear loose clothes that are made of material which allows your sweat to escape, or protect the areas with plasters.

Danger signs

Even the fittest athlete can rapidly develop health problems and you should always be conscious of how you are feeling. If, during or after your walk, you experience any of the following symptoms, stop and consult a doctor or medical expert as soon as possible:

- Chest pain or pressure
- Nausea
- Leg cramps or unsteadiness
- An unusually high heart rate
- Light-headedness or dizziness
- Shortness of breath
- Any other unusual discomfort.

Convert Your Steps Into Miles

Step Total

Step Length (see p 81)	1000	1500	2000	2500	3000	3500	4000	4500	5000	5500	6000	6500	7000	7500	8000	8500	9000	10000
12	.19	.28	.38	.47	.57	.66	.76	.85	.95	1.04	1.14	1.23	1.33	1.42	1.52	1.61	1.70	1.89
13	.21	.31	.41	.51	.62	.72	.82	.92	1.03	1.13	1.23	1.33	1.44	1.54	1.64	1.74	1.85	2.05
14	.22	.33	.44	.55	.66	.77	.88	.99	1.10	1.21	1.32	1.43	1.55	1.66	1.77	1.88	1.99	2.21
15	.24	.36	.47	.59	.71	.83	.95	1.07	1.18	1.30	1.42	1.54	1.66	1.78	1.89	2.01	2.13	2.37
16	.25	.38	.50	.63	.76	.88	1.01	1.14	1.26	1.39	1.51	1.64	1.77	1.89	2.02	2.14	2.27	2.52
17	.27	.40	.54	.67	.80	.94	1.07	1.21	1.34	1.47	1.61	1.74	1.88	2.01	2.15	2.28	2.41	2.68
18	.28	.43	.57	.71	.85	.99	1.14	1.28	1.42	1.56	1.70	1.85	1.99	2.13	2.27	2.41	2.56	2.84
19	.30	.45	.60	.75	.90	1.00	1.20	1.35	1.50	1.65	1.80	1.95	2.10	2.25	2.40	2.55	2.70	3.00
20	.32	.47	.63	.79	.95	1.10	1.26	1.42	1.58	1.74	1.89	2.05	2.21	2.37	2.53	2.68	2.84	3.16
21	.33	.50	.66	.83	.99	1.16	1.33	1.49	1.66	1.82	1.99	2.15	2.32	2.49	2.65	2.82	2.98	3.31
22	.35	.52	.69	.87	1.04	1.26	1.39	1.56	1.74	1.91	2.08	2.26	2.43	2.60	2.78	2.96	3.12	3.47
23	.36	.54	.73	.90	1.09	1.27	1.45	1.63	1.81	2.00	2.18	2.36	2.54	2.72	2.90	3.08	3.26	3.63
24	.38	.57	.76	.95	1.14	1.33	1.52	1.70	1.89	2.08	2.27	2.46	2.65	2.84	3.03	3.22	3.41	3.79
25	.39	.59	.79	.99	1.18	1.38	1.58	1.78	1.97	2.17	2.37	2.56	2.76	2.96	3.16	3.35	3.55	3.95
26	.41	.62	.82	1.03	1.23	1.44	1.64	1.85	2.05	2.26	2.46	2.67	2.87	3.08	3.28	3.49	3.70	4.10
27	.43	.64	.85	1.07	1.28	1.49	1.70	1.92	2.13	2.34	2.56	2.77	2.98	3.20	3.41	3.62	3.84	4.26
28	.44	.66	.88	1.10	1.33	1.55	1.77	1.99	2.21	2.43	2.65	2.87	3.10	3.31	3.54	3.76	3.98	4.42
29	.46	.69	.92	1.14	1.37	1.60	1.83	2.06	2.29	2.52	2.75	2.98	3.20	3.43	3.66	3.89	4.12	4.58
30	.47	.71	.95	1.18	1.42	1.66	1.89	2.13	2.37	2.60	2.84	3.08	3.31	3.55	3.79	4.02	4.26	4.73
31	.49	.73	.98	1.22	1.47	1.71	2.00	2.20	2.45	2.70	2.94	3.18	3.42	3.67	3.91	4.16	4.40	4.89
32	.51	.76	1.01	1.26	1.52	1.77	2.02	2.27	2.53	2.78	3.03	3.28	3.54	3.79	4.04	4.29	4.55	5.05
33	.52	.78	1.04	1.30	1.56	1.82	2.08	2.34	2.60	2.86	3.13	3.39	3.65	3.91	4.17	4.43	4.69	5.21
34	.54	.80	1.07	1.34	1.61	1.88	2.15	2.41	2.68	2.96	3.22	3.49	3.76	4.02	4.29	4.56	4.83	5.37
35	.55	.83	1.10	1.38	1.66	1.93	2.20	2.49	2.76	3.04	3.31	3.59	3.87	4.14	4.42	4.70	4.97	5.52
36	.57	.85	1.14	1.42	1.70	1.99	2.27	2.56	2.84	3.13	3.41	3.69	3.98	4.26	4.55	4.83	5.11	5.68

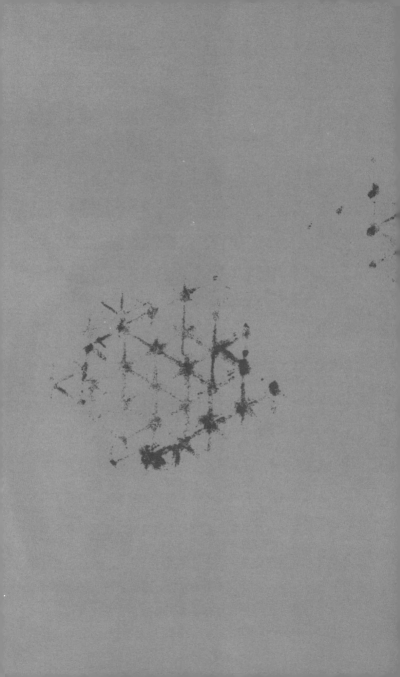

8 Walking off the Calories

"MY DOCTOR TOLD ME TO STOP HAVING INTIMATE DINNERS FOR FOUR. UNLESS THERE ARE THREE OTHER PEOPLE."

Orson Welles

Walking, food and calories

Many people turn to step counting as a new form of diet, an alternative to Dr Atkins, the GI diet, or any of the other currently fashionable weight-loss programmes. As a means of exercising, increasing your fitness and toning your muscles, "serious" walking will almost certainly help you lose weight, but not if you ignore the basic rules.

Very simply: if your aim is to lose a significant amount of weight, in particular excess body fat, then you must consume fewer calories (the energy value provided by food) than you burn off each day. How many calories you burn depends, generally, on your lifestyle and your size. An average woman will get through around 2,000 calories a day, and a man will expend about 2,500.

In order to lose weight effectively, you should aim to consume 500 fewer calories per day than your daily caloric needs. However, you must not go below 1,200 calories per day unless you are on a medically supervised weight loss programme or after consultation with your doctor.

TOP TIP

Instead of a morning coffee or tea break, take a walking break.

So you need to understand and reduce the calories in the food you are consuming and/or increase the amount you are burning. At last, we are back to walking. The further and faster you walk, the more calories you will use and if you are also controlling your calorie intake – hey presto! – the pounds should begin to disappear.

> ### Eight ways NOT to lose weight
>
> Skipping meals
> Magic diet pills
> Trying to lose it all in two weeks
> Fluid not food diets
> Dawdling
> Only eating one food
> Rushing your meals
> Cheating

Going the extra mile

To get your weight-loss programme really in gear, you will need to reconsider your walking. Are you reaching your 10,000-step goal every day? Are you going for at least one walk of over 20 minutes that leaves you slightly out of breath? Are you walking round office corridors and shopping malls, or are you taking steps and panting up hills? Now you have got to try to turn your steps into a proper exercise routine.

Distance remains the most important thing to us. Make sure you are hitting that 10,000 mark as often as possible and, whenever you can, are pushing on towards 12,000. Try also to increase your pace (remember though: quick steps, short strides) whenever you can. You can see

from the following chart what effect that can have on
your calorie expenditure.

Estimated calories burned per hour of walking			
Weight	Calories burned		
	4,000 sph*	6,000 sph	8,000 sph
120 lbs	160	215	280
210 lbs	210	285	375
265 lbs	265	360	470

* steps per hour

Effective walking

If you learn to vary your distance and speed, you can plan
your walking day or week much more easily. You might
decide to do a tough series of walks every other day and a
rest day once a week, or perhaps take a 15-minute
"intensive" walk once a day. You can tailor your
programme to suit your particular lifestyle. But before
you do this there are a number of other pointers that
might help you in a step-aided, weight-loss programme.

Take a walk first thing in the morning
You have less easy-to-burn carbohydrate fuel in your
bloodstream in the morning, so you're more likely
to burn stored fat.

Take a long walk daily
Walking briskly for 30 minutes burns more calories
than three 10-minute walks throughout the day.
"Continuous" walking burns about 60 more calories

per day than "intermittent" walking. The difference could amount to losing about 5 lbs a year.

Look at other ways of increasing the intensity of your walk
Head for the hills, avoid escalators and take the steps – anything to get that pulse moving a little faster.

Carry extra weight
But be careful not to add more than 10 lbs and do not carry anything that will alter your walking technique and posture. Carry excess weight in a backpack or wear weighted wrist bands that are available at good sports shops.

Did You Know?

Although you burn fewer calories by walking for an hour than running for an hour, walking can be better for someone wishing to lose weight. When you run a mile, you're burning mostly sugar, or carbohydrates, which gives your body fast energy in bursts. When you walk a mile, your metabolism has time to switch from burning carbohydrates to burning fat.

Healthy eating – the basics

It is always important to eat the right kind of foods, but if you are taking regular exercise and want to lose weight, this becomes even more essential. If you are

willing to put in the
right amount of work
on the streets and
lanes and eat sensibly –
cutting out fatty foods,
pastries, chips, beer
and chocolate – you
should be able to lose
at least a pound a
month. This is slow

TOP TIP

Freeze water in your
water bottle. It will melt
slowly while you walk
so that you'll have a
constant supply of cold,
refreshing water.

weight loss, but you will be losing fat not water, and
it's really the only way to lose it permanently. Keep it
up for six months and not only should you have lost
around half a stone but you will have gone a long way
towards changing your body shape and to changing
over to a long-term healthy lifestyle.

Each day should include:

- Four small (or two larger) servings of meat, fish or
  poultry (or a veggie alternative, such as tofu)
- At least three servings of vegetables and two
  servings of fruits
- Five servings of bread or rice, preferably
  wholemeal or brown
- Two servings of low-fat or non-fat dairy products,
  i.e. milk, yoghurt, cottage cheese or reduced-fat
  cheese

Dietary dos and don'ts

Do eat six small meals a day – breakfast, lunch, dinner and three snacks.

Do ensure your diet is made up of 50 per cent carbohydrate (bread, fruit, rice, pasta, vegetables), 25 per cent protein (meat, fish and eggs) and 25 per cent unsaturated fats (oily fish, nuts, seeds).

Do boil or grill your food whenever possible. If you have to use oil, use olive oil.

Do drink lots of water. Often you think you are hungry when you are actually thirsty. Drinking with a meal will also help you eat less.

Do eat more slowly. Taste each mouthful before you swallow and you will find you need less.

Don't deny yourself treats completely. Turning down that glass of wine, bar of chocolate, a piece of a friend's birthday cake will eventually lead to you caving in. Allow yourself a treat now and then – and walk off the extra calories – then return to your programme.

Don't skip meals or certain elements of your diet (such as carbohydrates). If you do, you will become listless and unable to complete or even start your walk.

Don't eat too big a portion. Maintaining portion control is important. One serving should contain a medium-sized potato or a few tablespoons of pasta, about 4 oz (120 g) vegetables and a small piece of meat or fish.

Don't fill up on fruit. Some fruits such as bananas and pineapples are high in calories and sugar. Have your regular five servings of fruit and vegetables a day, but try not to overdo things.

Eating for walking

The above dietary advice should enable you to undergo a reasonably active walking programme without leaving you feeling weak or sluggish. There are, however, a few tips that you might find useful if you are planning long or very rigorous walks:

- Balance carbohydrates and proteins at every meal to ensure a continuous energy level.
- Take drinking water to sip periodically as you walk. Dehydration is the main reason for exhaustion.
- If you are taking a snack in order to refuel en route, choose an apple or a banana, a dried fruit mix or perhaps some pumpkin seeds..
- Even if you are not feeling especially hungry, have a light meal two or three hours before a walk which will last over two hours.

Simple or complex?

Carbohydrates are the main source of glucose, the body's preferred energy source. They are found in vegetables, fruit and grain products such as bread and pasta. But some carbohydrates act differently to others and it can be helpful to know which ones to consume when you are exercizing hard.

> **TOP TIP**
> Sign up for a sponsored charity walk and help others, while you are helping yourself.

Complex carbohydrates

Complex carbohydrates provide slow-release energy over a long period, limiting the amount of sugar converted into fat. This makes them ideal to take a few hours prior to a strenuous walk. As long as you remember to eat them in moderate portions, these foods will should fit in easily with your daily diet:

Pasta

Brown rice

Potatoes

Other root vegetables

Wholemeal, granary and brown breads

High-fibre breakfast cereals

Porridge oats, or Weetabix, or shredded wheat cereals

Swedish-style crispbread

Muesli

Oatcakes

Peas, beans and lentils

Simple carbohydrates

Sugar and other simple carbohydrates release quick energy, which as you might suppose is used up just as quickly by the body. If you are about to set out for a walk but don't feel you have the right energy levels, or you have returned and are feeling hungry and lethargic, the following foods can provide a pick-me-up and should still fit into your daily diet.

Apples
Blackcurrants
Grapefruit
Kiwi fruit
Oranges
Pears
Strawberries

When you are engaging in a regular exercise routine, you are increasing your basal metabolic rate – the number of calories you burn each day at rest. Even when you are sleeping, you will be working off the calories much more effectively.

A stepper's day

Breakfast

If you do your main walk first thing in the morning, you may not want to eat beforehand. To reduce unnecessary strain on your body, avoid going from sleeping to walking in less than half an hour. Use the first part of that half hour to drink a glass of water

and eat a slice of bread or toast. Anything spread
on the toast should be spread very sparingly.
Then do some gentle warming up before you start on
your walk. When you finish, have something
else for breakfast – bran flakes, a grapefruit or a
low-fat yoghurt. If your walk takes you over to your
place of work, try to take something with you to
have when you finish.

> ### Did You Know?
> You lose weight while you sleep.

Lunch

If you do a lunchtime walk, don't miss lunch. Keep
it for when you return – it'll give you something to look
forward to when you feel as if you want to give up.
Try having a salad with plenty of ingredients, swapping
them round over the week.

Dinner

If you walk in the afternoon or early evening, you may
be able to follow your walk with your evening meal.
If you finish your walk some time before your meal,
have a light snack immediately afterwards so that your
muscles can refuel while they are most
receptive to doing so. If you walk after your meal,
remember to leave it as long as possible as before you
start or you may hamper the digestion process. Keep

your supper light to avoid causing drowsiness and save some fruit for when you return.

Motivational meals

Rules are there to be broken. If breaking them can motivate you, then "harness" this as a reward for a session you might otherwise have missed. Better to treat yourself to that fried egg or bar of chocolate than to give up the routine.

> **TOP TIP**
> Most serious walkers notice favourable changes to their body weight and shape in about four to eight weeks.

Watch your step!

Thinking of treating yourself? Here's how many steps it will cost you!

Drinks	
Tea or coffee with semi-skimmed milk	350
Glass of white wine	2,175
Glass of red wine	3,125
Can of cola	3,475
Pint of lager	4,075
Gin and tonic	5,000

Snack attack

Cinema carton of salted popcorn	3,025
Chocolate wafer biscuit	3,050
Packet of crisps	4,500
Plain bagel	4,875
Doughnut	5,250
Latte with full-fat milk	6500
Snickers bar	7,775
Toast, jam and butter (two rounds)	8,550
Cheese and pickle sandwich	10,500
Blueberry muffin	10,400
Large fish and chips	15,000
Roast beef, carrots, sprouts and roast potatoes	15,775
Sweet 'n' sour with special fried rice	27,500
Eight-inch pepperoni pizza	36,250
French fries	5,000
Chocolate ice cream (small portion)	4,500

Healthy eating

Small carrot	45
Tomato	350
Apple	2000
Orange	1,475
One ounce of cheddar cheese	2,300
Green salad with french dressing	3,050
Banana	3,125
Pot of fruit yoghurt	3,275
Can of baked beans	3,875
Portion of roast chicken (no skin)	4,150
Baked potato	4,950
Bowl of cornflakes with skimmed milk	5,000

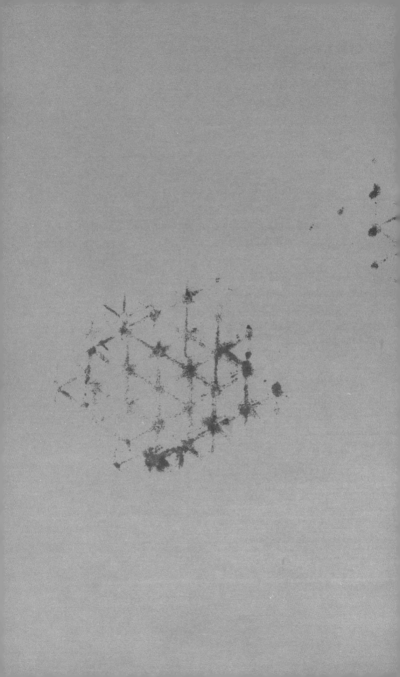

9 When the going gets tough...

"WILL YOU WALK A LITTLE FASTER SAID A WHITING TO A SNAIL." ALICE'S ADVENTURES IN WONDERLAND, Lewis Carroll

No matter how enthusiastically you take to step counting, there will come a time when you'll wonder if it is really worth it. It might be after nine months' enjoyable striding on the city streets or it could be after four days' miserable plodding down muddy lanes. Perhaps you've had a week's holiday and have lost the routine... Maybe the nights are getting colder and darker and there are fewer repeats on TV... Or it could be that you are just sick of the whole walking business and are about to throw those trainers, with some force, into the rubbish bin. Wait...

Think back to why you started step counting. The chances are that you haven't achieved your aim yet. And if you are satisfied with your progress, why stop now? Reflect on the good moments: when you realized that you could get into a smaller-sized pair of jeans, when you met the good-looking person out walking their dog, or when you eased into that bath with every ounce of your body aching and got out an hour later feeling wonderful.

And finally, remember... only losers quit

If you are bored with your routine

Change things around
Swap morning for evening walks. Vary the distance; if you were doing a few short walks a day, try stepping out for one longer workout – and vice versa.

Did You Know?

Walking sideways burns 78 per cent more calories than walking forwards.

Investigate new areas in which to walk

You'll be amazed at what you'll find of interest even in the seemingly dullest of industrial environments.

Use a portable music player

Walkmans, iPods and radios can all be carried easily while you walk (see page 113 for a step speeder's Top 20 tunes). And, you don't have to listen to music – there is a massive selection of audio books that are available as well. Be careful not to turn the volume up too loud so that it stops you hearing traffic and other dangers.

Introduce an element of competition

Find someone to race against – if one of you is much better than the other, then find a handicap system that evens things out; for example, let them start five minutes before you. If you are on your own, start racing against the clock. See how many steps you can do in 15 minutes and then try to beat your own record. Or just time yourself on your regular route and try to finish quicker each time.

Swap some other exercise with parts of your walking schedule

Swimming, cycling and aerobics classes will all help you work off the calories. If you want to count these exercises as steps, calculate the step equivalent by using the following chart:

Approximate step-per-minute equivalents for non-walking activities

Rates described here will vary according to the rigour of the individual exercise.

Sports	
Badminton	98
Cycling (leisurely)	51
Cycling (moderate)	93
Cycling (fast)	130
Football	144
Golf	131
Horse riding (leisurely)	31
Ice skating	84
Roller skating	150
Rowing (leisurely)	147
Running, 10 mph (6 min/mile)	463
Running, 8 mph (7.5 min mile)	391
Running, 6 mph (10 min mile)	290
Running, 5 mph (12 min/mile)	232
Skipping (about 150 turns/min)	167
Squash	198
Swimming (treading water)	49
Swimming (breast stroke at 1 MPH)	89
Swimming (crawl at 1 MPH)	91
Swimming (backstroke at 1 MPH)	111
Table tennis	116
Tennis (doubles)	102
Tennis (singles)	232

Around the house

Fetching and carrying (over 15 lbs)	176
Gardening (light)	73
Gardening (general)	96
Gardening (heavy digging)	278
House painting	78
Housework (scrubbing the floor)	110
Housework (vacuuming)	101
Housework (washing windows)	87
Mowing lawn (manual)	122
Mowing lawn (power)	109
Stair climbing (slow)	90
Stair climbing (moderate)	180
Stair climbing (fast)	267
Washing the car	131

Classes

Aerobics (low impact)	118
Aerobic (workout)	140
Circuit training	240
Dancing	93
Kickboxing	290
Pilates	160
Step	280
Trampoline	101

Give yourself a break

Perhaps take a week off, or even two. But put a date in the diary to remind you of when you are going to start again and make sure you stick to it.

If it is getting dark, wet and cold

Kit yourself out properly
In decent waterproofs – a jacket with a hood, trousers and shoes (you can even buy waterproof overshoes) – a walk in the rain is a completely different experience. Similarly, if it is cold, wear layers so that you remain comfortable throughout the walk. Warm up well indoors before you set off, so that you will not need to take a heavy coat just for those first few minutes. And if it is dark, you'll feel safer dressed in reflective clothing and carrying a torch.

Find an indoor route you can take
Be imaginative. You may be lucky enough to work in a large office with a few storeys. Devise a route that will take you up, down and around the whole building. Perhaps there is a heated shopping centre where you can happily walk around for 30 minutes or more.

Join a gym
Nearly all gyms will have a treadmill where you can happily stroll away your steps. You might find others who can help keep you motivated. You never know, you might even find some of the other fitness equipment interesting enough to try.

As a last resort – ease off on the outdoor walking
Continue to do as many indoor steps as you can and, as mentioned above, try substituting another form of indoor exercise for some of your steps. But, again, put a

date in your diary when the weather begins to improve and make sure, when that day comes, that you are out clocking up those steps.

> **TOP TIP**
> Get yourself a dog and start to enjoy those "walkies".

If you are not losing weight

Persevere
If you have followed the healthy eating and step-counting advice in the book, you should be able to lose weight. This is not a crash diet, so it might be a month or more before you notice any weight loss. Don't give up too soon.

Are you cheating with your eating?
Take a note of everything you consume and tally up your calories. You might be forgetting that mid-morning latte or could it be you are a little generous with your portions?

Are you regularly clocking up your target number of steps?
Are you hitting 10,000 yet? If the answer to these questions is yes, you will have to consider upping your target. People have varying metabolic rates (the time it takes to burn calories) and if you are unlucky you may have to do more steps than the average person.

How much time are you spending walking at your target heart rate (see pane belowl)?

This is the essential part for those wishing to lose weight. Stop dawdling, start working up a little sweat and you should begin to see some results.

Target Heart Rate

To know if you are training at the right pace work out your Target Heart Rate by subtracting your age from 226 (220 for men) to calculate your Maximum Heart Rate (MHR).

Warm-up zone – 50–60 per cent of maximum heart rate

This is the rate beginners should exercise at and more experienced walkers should use to warm up. Even at this rate, your exercise can help decrease body fat – 85 per cent of calories burned in this zone are fats – high blood pressure and cholesterol.

Fat-burning zone – 61–70 per cent of maximum heart rate

Although still burning 85 per cent fat calories, this exercise rate is more intense and burns more total calories.

Aerobic zone – 71–80 per cent of maximum heart rate

As well as burning more calories (50 per cent from fat) this zone will build stamina, improving the strength of your heart and lungs.

Anaerobic zone – 81–90 per cent of maximum heart rate

This is a high-intensity zone burning more calories (15 per cent from fat). You will only be able to stay in this zone for short periods but the longer and more frequently you manage to reach this level, the better..

Red-line zone – 91–100 per cent of maximum heart rate

Although this zone burns the highest number of calories, it is only for the very fittest of walkers because it is incredibly intense and can be dangerous.

Stepping up the pace

As most people these days are pushed for time, it is much easier for them to speed up their walk than to walk longer distances. However, knowing when and how much to increase the pace is sometimes difficult. With reference to your Target Heart Rate (see page 110), you should be aiming to spend as much time as possible in the Fat-Burning Zone (see page 110), stepping up where possible to the Aerobic

> **TOP TIP**
> Schedule time for a walk in your diary and underline it as a priority engagement!

Zone and above. How long you spend in each zone depends on your fitness. A beginner might spend only a few minutes of a 20-minute walk above 50 per cent of their MHR, whereas an experienced walker should be looking to spend the majority of the time pushing 75 per cent and only dropping off for a breather here and there.

Target Heart Rate

Age	Target Zone (beats per minute, 60-75% of maximum)	Average Maximum Heart Rate
20	120–150	200
25	117–146	195
30	114–142	190
35	111–138	185
40	108–135	180
45	105–131	175
50	102–127	170
55	99–123	165
60	96–120	160
65	93–116	155
70	90–113	150

Interval training

Beginners should always start with interval training, until they build up their fitness. This involves increasing your pace and holding it there for a set time or until you can hold it no longer. You then return to your normal pace until you feel ready to increase it again. For example, walk for two minutes at around 2,000 steps an hour (about 65 steps in total), then walk for one minute at 3,000 steps an hour (about 50 steps), return to the slower pace for another two minutes and then step it up again. Until the end of the walk, you should never be too exhausted to maintain the slower pace. And, as time goes on, you should find yourself recovering more quickly and be able to spend more time at the faster pace.

DID YOU KNOW?

In Japan, an average household has 3.1 pedometers.

Walk the Beat

If it is safe to do so where you are walking, listening to music – on an iPod or a Walkman – as you walk can spur you on. Pick something with a uptempo beat and with a bit of a zip in it. Just for fun, here's a Top 20 to inspire you, but obviously the choice is yours. Just don't choose something that will have you doing the funeral march!

'Little Less Conversation' – Elvis Presley
'Lose My Breath' – Destiny's Child
'Walk This Way' – Run DMC and Aerosmith
'Disco Inferno' – The Tramps

'Don't Stop 'Til You Get Enough' – Michael Jackson
'The Heat Is On' – Glenn Frey
'Walk The Dinosaur' – Was Not Was
'The Only Way Is Up' – Yazz
'Jump' – Van Halen (or Sister Sledge)
'Wanna Be Startin Something' – Michael Jackson
'Wake Me Up Before You Go Go' – Wham!
'Into The Groove' – Madonna
'Roll With It' – Oasis
'Rhythm Is A Dancer' - Snap
'Start Me Up' – The Rolling Stones
'Holding Out For A Hero' – Bonnie Tyler
'Leader Of The Pack' – The Shangri-Las
'I Want to Break Free' – Queen
'Jenny From The Block' – Jennifer Lopez
'Love Train' – The O'Jays

Dehydration – a warning

If you are starting to work harder on your walks, remember not to get dehydrated. The average person can lose as much as 0.5–1 litre of fluid during an hour of exercise. This in turn can lead to a 20 per cent reduction in athletic performance because strength, power and breathing are all affected. Unfortunately, your body will not show signs of dehydration until it's too late. When the thirst hits, you will already be severely dehydrated. Then, you will stop feeling thirsty after your first sip and often not drink enough. Therefore, you must learn to detect the signs and take precautions.

Signs of dehydration

- Increased thirst
- Dry mouth
- Fatigue
- Dizziness
- Light-headedness
- Palpitations (feeling that the heart is jumping or pounding)
- Confusion
- Sluggishness
- An inability to sweat
- A decreased urine output or, if urine is concentrated, it will be a deeply yellow or amber colour

Tips on hydrating

- Start the day off with a glass of water.
- Drink throughout the day (every 15–20 minutes).
- Carry a water bottle when walking and drink 8 fl ozs of water every 15 minutes.
- Before and after an intense walk, try an isotonic sports drink.
- Compensate for fluid losses due to caffeine, alcohol, exercise intensity, and weather.
- If you are walking for over an hour and find yourself sweating, switch to a sports drink after the first hour to replace salt – or eat a snack that has some salt.

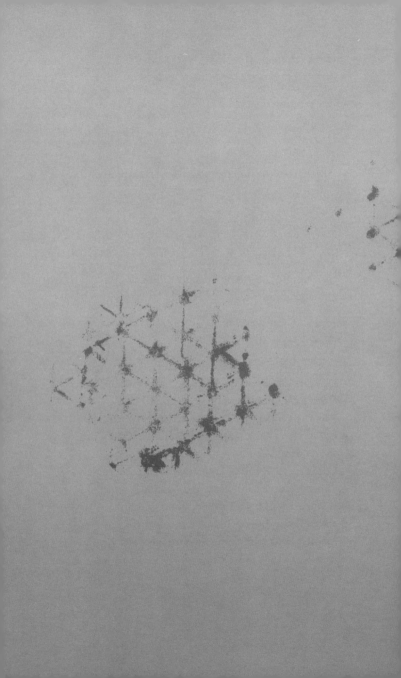

10 Going for the Burn

"A MAN'S HEALTH CAN BE JUDGED BY WHICH HE TAKES TWO AT A TIME — PILLS OR STAIRS." Joan Welsh

So you have really caught the bug. You are mastering your 10,000 steps with ease and are walking at a pace you feel is doing you good. What next? Well, if you are fit enough – and, if in doubt, you should check with your doctor to make sure you are – there are some exciting options open to you.

Hitting the 20,000 mark

If you are serious about joining the pedometer "pros", you could consider upping your step tally to 20,000. This is serious walking, so you need to prepare yourself a little more thoroughly.

- Invest in quality sporting equipment that feels light and makes you feel comfortable.
- Don't try to increase your target too much too soon. Increases should be at 10 per cent a week.
- On 20,000 steps you will probably lose weight. Is this your aim? If not, up your calorie intake accordingly or try some diluted carbo-loading powder (available in good sports stores).
- Remember the advice on avoiding dehydration (see page 114).

Exerstriding/Nordic walking

Try taking the skills you have built up from your step-counting walks even further. Exerstriding, also known as "pole walking", "fitness walking" or "Nordic walking", has been gaining in popularity around the world, especially in Scandinavia, since the late 1980s. Basically fitness walking with specially designed poles, it maximises the benefits gained from step counting. Burning 20–70 per cent more calories, it also strengthens arms, shoulder, back and those important "core strength" trunk muscles, taking pain and injury-causing stresses off your hips, knees and feet.

For more information visit the International Nordic Walking Association at inwa.nordicwalking.com/

or contact:

> Nordic Walking Association for Great Britain
> and Ireland
> Nordic Health Ltd
> PO Box 49009
> London N11 1YX
>
> Nordic Walking USA
> 2619 2nd Street
> Suite 4
> Santa Monica
> CA 90405

Walking the marathon

If you are looking for a real challenge, how about walking a marathon? First, bear in mind that it is 26. 2 miles. That's somewhere in the region of 52,000 steps and it will take you anything from 6 to 12 hours depending on your fitness. You will need to be fit to begin with – perhaps you have already walked some half-marathons – and be ready to commit around three months to some serious training during which you will regularly be clocking up 20–30,000-step walks. The chances of injury are quite high and you will need to apply successfully to the organizers to take part, especially for the popular London, New York and Paris Marathons. Having said all that, people of all ages and physical conditions have succeeded and enjoyed marathon walking.

For further information visit:
www.marathonwalking.com

DID YOU KNOW?

You need to use 200 muscles in your body to walk.

Race walking

If you feel you have a special talent for walking fast, you may wish to move into the competitive arena.
Race walking has been an Olympic sport for 100 years with race distances of 20 and 50 kilometres for men and 20 kilometres for women. A beginner would need to start clocking up about 2,000 steps in 15 minutes so as not to be embarrassed by the competition.

Race walking has a specific technique, but if you are walking using the technique advised in this book, then you shouldn't need to adapt your style too much. There are two main rules to competitive walking and they are:

1 You must be in contact with the ground at all times.
2 The knee of the supporting leg must stay straight from the time of foot contact with the ground until the next leg passes under the body.

Further information is available at:
www.racewalkingassociation.btinternet.co.uk
www.usaracewalking.com

Hill walking

Those who have particularly enjoyed tackling the hills during their walks, might consider focusing their efforts vertically. Hill walking can be done in the course of a day or over a week or more and if you take part in it you can either camp, or stay in a hostel or hotel overnight. It can be very strenuous and you should think about investing in walking boots. But the rewards can be spectacular – incredible views, great exercise and a chance to get away from it all.

For more information visit:
www.hillwalking.org.uk

Gadgets

The pedometer is an incredible, but simple gadget that has revolutionized people's attitudes to walking. If you have the bug and want to invest further, here are a few other technological advances that might help you.

Advanced pedometers

The pedometer that usually comes with this book is all you need to count your steps, but if you have the money, there are a host of other pedometers on the market that will provide other information. Among the facilities they can provide are:

- Measurement of your stride and calculation of total distance walked
- Calculation BMI and Body Fat Level
- Assessment of your progress towards step targets
- Measurement of calories burned
- Some even include a built-in FM radio!

Heart-rate monitors

While taking your own pulse is not usually a problem, it is much easier to glance down at your wrist and see a reading. Monitoring your heart rate involves strapping a small wireless transmitter to your chest. This sends a signal to a monitor display on your wrist, which is able to display your pulse rate, and more, at the press of a button. Like pedometers, they can also feature a range of related facilities.

The less expensive pulsemeter is a similar, if simpler, gadget. Carried in a pocket or worn around your neck, it has an infrared sensor over which you can place your finger for a heart-rate reading.

Treadmills

Those with a particular dislike of everything the outside world can throw at them and who have a spare bit of cash – around the £1,000 mark – might consider a home treadmill. You'll need a fair amount of space as it isn't a compact piece of equipment, but it does mean you'll be able to walk whenever you choose – in front of the TV or with the stereo blasting.

Many treadmills have arm rests, these are useful for keeping our balance when first using the machine, but can be too much of a temptation to tired steppers. Walkers should remember their technique, swing their arms and try to keep a straight back.

The readout on modern treadmills will enable you to change your speed and keep a check on the distance you have walked. Most decent and state-of-the-art machines will also allow you to increase the gradient up to around 10 per cent. As we have seen, this is particularly useful for those aiming at weight loss.

If you are thinking of buying a treadmill, be sure to try it out first. The showroom should help you, but it is a good idea to take a free or reduced-price trial at a gym and see how happy you feel on the apparatus.

TOP TIP

Always eat breakfast, even if it is a piece of fruit on your way out of the door.

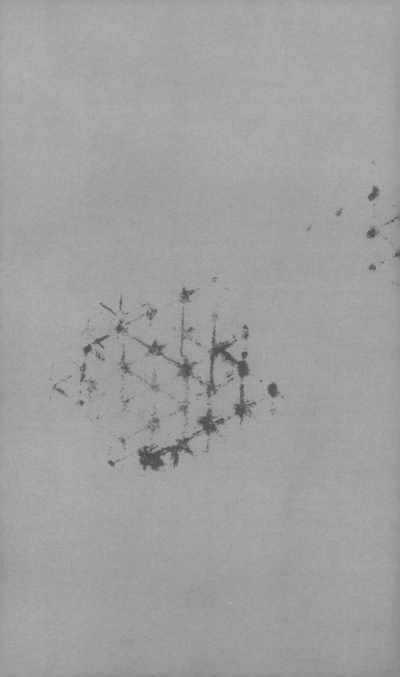

Walking Log

These pages have been designed for you to fill in and keep details of your own walking progress. Remember, how hard you push yourself is up to you. Even if it takes a year to progress to the 10,000-steps-a-day mark, it will be worth it and you will be doing yourself a power of good along the way.

Don't feel you have to fill in every single piece of information every day, but the more details you manage to record, the more complete the picture of your progress that emerges will be.

There is space for the following information:

Step Target
- Be aware of how many steps you currently take in a day before setting a target.
- Be realistic. Set a target you believe you are able to reach.
- Never increase your target by more than 10 per cent a week.
- If you are struggling to reach your target, don't be afraid to decrease the total and build up again.

Steps Walked
- Remember to wear your pedometer from socks on to socks off – from first thing in the morning until last thing at night.
- Take your reading when you take the pedometer off at night.
- Compare your total with your target. If you are below it, you might wish to make up the difference tomorrow. If you are ahead, you could award yourself an easy day.

Weekly total so far
- It is perfectly acceptable to count your weekly rather than your daily steps.
- Make sure you are not leaving yourself too much to do at the end of the week.

Intensity
- Try to note down any time during your walks where you might have exceeded 50 per cent of your maximum heart rate
- As you progress, try to increase the intensity of at least one reasonable walk over 10 minutes.

Calorie intake
- If you are aiming for weight loss, you may wish to note down your calorie intake for the day – accurately, or by rule of thumb.

Calories burned
- Refer to the chart on page 92 to estimate the amount of calories you may have burned throughout the day. Remember to add the 2,000 (2,500 for men) that you expend through normal activity.

Walks 5–10 minutes
Walks 10–20 minutes
Walks over 20 minutes

- Try to note the approximate number of steps you took in one walk. This will help you work out whether you are getting sufficient exercise from your step total.
- Unless you are very unfit or a complete beginner, you should be looking to do at least one walk of over 20 minutes and one of over 10.

Notes
- Jot down any aches and pains or tips and tricks you may have discovered to help you reach your target.
- Note how many steps you can do if you get off the bus a stop early, how many stairs there are to the top of your office building, or even which parts of a walk you find interesting, challenging or easy to build up speed.
- Keep a record of any interesting sights or thoughts you might have experienced on your walks!

Week One

Thought for the week

ACHIEVEMENT IS LARGELY THE
PRODUCT OF STEADILY RAISING ONE'S
LEVELS OF ASPIRATION – Jack Nicklaus

No matter how fit you believe yourself to be, take it easy in
the first week. Remember we are aiming for slow progress.
Try to be as consistent as you can over the week, reaching
roughly the same target each day.

- If you are a beginner, you should be aiming to do 4–5,000
  steps each day this week.
- If you are an intermediate ,or are aiming for weight loss,
  try for 5–6,000 steps each day this week.
- If you consider yourself fairly fit, try to do at least 6,000
  steps each day this week.

Try to get into a routine as soon as possible. You don't need
to stick to it rigidly but it will reassure you that you can
make the total every day. Perhaps try to get three-quarters of
the steps completed before the evening meal and then take
an evening walk to complete the day's total or, if you have
time, have a long walk in the afternoon when you can
complete a large amount of the total in one go.

   If you are trying to lose weight, start by cutting out the
things you know you shouldn't have – chocolate, chips,
excess alcohol – you know what they are!

Monday

Date: ....

Step target: ....

Steps walked: ....

Weekly total so far: ....

Intensity: ....

Calorie intake: ....

Calories burned: ....

Notes: ....

....

....

Thought for the day

YOU HAVE BRAINS IN YOUR HEAD, YOU
HAVE FEET IN YOUR SHOES. YOU CAN
STEER YOURSELF IN ANY DIRECTION
YOU CHOOSE – Dr Seuss

Tuesday

Date: ....

Step target: ....

Steps walked: ....

Weekly total so far: ....

Intensity: ....

Calorie intake: ....

Calories burned: ....

Notes: ....

....

....

Thought for the day

FALL DOWN SEVEN TIMES, STAND UP
EIGHT TIMES – Japanese proverb

Wednesday

Date: ....

Step target: ....

Steps walked: ....

Weekly total so far: ....

Intensity: ....

Calorie intake: ....

Calories burned: ....

Notes: ....

....

....

Thought for the day

HAPPINESS IS A STATE OF ACTIVITY –

Aristotle

Thursday

Date: ....

Step target: ....

Steps walked: ....

Weekly total so far: ....

Intensity: ....

Calorie intake: ....

Calories burned: ....

Notes: ....

....

....

Friday

Date: ....

Step target: ....

Steps walked: ....

Weekly total so far: ....

Intensity: ....

Calorie intake: ....

Calories burned: ....

Notes: ....

....

....

Thought for the day

EITHER YOU RUN THE DAY, OR THE DAY
RUNS YOU – Jim Rohn

Saturday

Date: ....

Step target: ....

Steps walked: ....

Weekly total so far: ....

Intensity: ....

Calorie intake: ....

Calories burned: ....

Notes: ....

....

....

Thought for the day

YOUR THOUGHTS ARE THE ARCHITECTS
OF YOUR DESTINY – David O McKay

Sunday

Date: ....

Step target: ....

Steps walked: ....

Weekly total so far: ....

Intensity: ....

Calorie intake: ....

Calories burned: ....

Notes: ....

....

....

Thought for the day

GREAT CHANGES MAY NOT HAPPEN
RIGHT AWAY, BUT WITH EFFORT EVEN
THE DIFFICULT MAY BECOME EASY
– Bill Blackman

Week Two

SUCCESS IS THE RESULT OF SMALL

EFFORTS, REPEATED DAY IN, DAY OUT

– Robert J Collier

Look back over last week's tallies. Were you making your target comfortably? If so, you are ready to move on. If not, don't worry; stick to last week's targets, there is plenty of time to build up the step count. You may have been feeling a little achey after last week's exertions – that's OK; the pain should disappear over the next week.

- If you are a beginner, you should be aiming to do 4,500–5,500 steps each day this week.
- If you are an intermediate or are aiming for weight loss, try for 5,600–6,600 steps each day this week.
- If you consider yourself fairly fit, try to do at least 6,600 steps each day this week.

Consider how you made your total. You may have found it difficult to reach it in very small journeys like trips to the next floor at the office and have been left with a lot to make up after work. Or did you find it impossible to make time for a longish walk and rely on 10-minute stretches here and there? Carry on working out what is good for you and realizing how flexible your lifestyle enables you to be.

In the notes section, continue to record how you are making up the totals, but also try to jot down how you feel on and after each walk of any distance. Although we are not immediately concerned with getting more than steps out of our walk, it will be of interest later on in the programme.

Weight watchers may find it useful to record their weight or any other measurement at this point as, depending on your progress, you might hope to see some improvements in the weeks ahead. This week, attempt to up your vegetable and fruit intake to four or five portions a day.

Monday

Date: ....

Step target: ....

Steps walked: ....

Weekly total so far: ....

Intensity: ....

Calorie intake: ....

Calories burned: ....

Notes: ....

....

....

Thought for the day

WHERESOEVER YOU GO, GO WITH ALL
YOUR HEART – Confucius

Tuesday

Monday

Date: ....

Step target: ....

Steps walked: ....

Weekly total so far: ....

Intensity: ....

Calorie intake: ....

Calories burned: ....

Notes: ....

....

....

Thought for the day

DISCIPLINE IS THE BRIDGE BETWEEN GOALS AND ACCOMPLISHMENT

– Jim Rohn

Wednesday

Date: ....

Step target: ....

Steps walked: ....

Weekly total so far: ....

Intensity: ....

Calorie intake: ....

Calories burned: ....

Notes: ....

....

....

Thought for the day

HAPPINESS IS NOT A STATION YOU
ARRIVE AT BUT A MANNER OF
TRAVELLING – Margaret B Runbeck

Thursday

Date: ....

Step target: ....

Steps walked: ....

Weekly total so far: ....

Intensity: ....

Calorie intake: ....

Calories burned: ....

Notes: ....

....

....

Friday

Date: ....

Step target: ....

Steps walked: ....

Weekly total so far: ....

Intensity: ....

Calorie intake: ....

Calories burned: ....

Notes: ....
....
....

Thought for the day

EVER TRIED. EVER FAILED. NO MATTER.

TRY AGAIN, FAIL AGAIN, FAIL BETTER

– Samuel Beckett

Saturday

Date: ....

Step target: ....

Steps walked: ....

Weekly total so far: ....

Intensity: ....

Calorie intake: ....

Calories burned: ....

Notes: ....
....
....

Thought for the day

WHEN WE QUIET THE MIND, THE
SYMPHONY BEGINS – Anon

Sunday

Date: ....

Step target: ....

Steps walked: ....

Weekly total so far: ....

Intensity: ....

Calorie intake: ....

Calories burned: ....

Notes: ....

....

....

Thought for the day

FESTINA LENTE ("HASTEN SLOWLY")

– Suetonis

Week Three

Thought for the week

BOTH TEARS AND SWEAT ARE SALTY, BUT THEY RENDER A DIFFERENT RESULT. TEARS WILL GET YOU SYMPATHY; SWEAT WILL GET YOU CHANGE –

Reverend Jesse Jackson

Once again, don't move on to the new targets unless you feel comfortable managing last week's totals. If you have been walking every day, you should begin to feel a little fitter now. The longer walks should not take so much out of you and you might find you are sleeping better. Your body should be getting used to it by now and hopefully any aches you had have disappeared.

- If you are a beginner, you should be aiming to do 5,000–6,100 steps each day this week.
- If you are an intermediate, or are aiming for weight loss, try for 6,100–7,200 steps each day this week.
- If you consider yourself fairly fit, try to do at least 7,200 steps each day this week.

As the targets get higher, you may well find it more difficult to find the time to do them. If you haven't already, now is the time to work out when you can fit in one walk a day of at least 20 minutes. This will be the walk where you can concentrate most on getting yourself in shape.

Those trying to lose weight should stick with it. It is quite possible you haven't lost any weight yet, but what you have done is put in some vital foundations.

Monday

Date: ....

Step target: ....

Steps walked: ....

Weekly total so far: ....

Intensity: ....

Calorie intake: ....

Calories burned: ....

Notes: ....

....

....

Thought for the day

FAIR IS FOUL AND FOUL IS FAIR; HOVER
THROUGH THE FOG AND FILTHY AIR
– William Shakespeare

Tuesday

Date: ....

Step target: ....

Steps walked: ....

Weekly total so far: ....

Intensity: ....

Calorie intake: ....

Calories burned: ....

Notes: ....

....

....

Thought for the day

IF EXERCISE COULD BE PACKED IN A
PILL, IT WOULD BE THE SINGLE MOST
WIDELY PRESCRIBED AND BENEFICIAL
MEDICINE – US Institute on Aging

Wednesday

Date: ....

Step target: ....

Steps walked: ....

Weekly total so far: ....

Intensity: ....

Calorie intake: ....

Calories burned: ....

Notes: ....

....

....

Thought for the day

TWENTY YEARS FROM NOW YOU WILL BE
MORE DISAPPOINTED BY THE THINGS
YOU DIDN'T DO THAN THE THINGS YOU
DID – Mark Twain

Thursday

Date: ....

Step target: ....

Steps walked: ....

Weekly total so far: ....

Intensity: ....

Calorie intake: ....

Calories burned: ....

Notes: ....

....

....

Thought for the day

**THE LESS EFFORT, THE FASTER AND
MORE POWERFUL YOU WILL BE**

– Bruce Lee

Friday

Date: ....

Step target: ....

Steps walked: ....

Weekly total so far: ....

Intensity: ....

Calorie intake: ....

Calories burned: ....

Notes: ....
....
....

Thought for the day

IF YOU ARE DOING YOUR BEST, YOU
WILL NOT WORRY ABOUT FAILURE
– Robert Hillyer

Saturday

Date: ....

Step target: ....

Steps walked: ....

Weekly total so far: ....

Intensity: ....

Calorie intake: ....

Calories burned: ....

Notes: ....
....
....

Thought for the day

THE AIM OF LIFE IS TO LIVE, AND TO
LIVE IS TO BE AWARE – Henry Miller

Sunday

Date: ....

Step target: ....

Steps walked: ....

Weekly total so far: ....

Intensity: ....

Calorie intake: ....

Calories burned: ....

Notes: ....

....

....

Thought for the day

THE REAL VOYAGE OF DISCOVERY
CONSISTS NOT IN SEEKING NEW
LANDSCAPES, BUT IN SEEING WITH
NEW EYES – Marcel Proust

Week Four

AN EARLY MORNING WALK IS A BLESSING FOR THE WHOLE DAY

– Henry D Thoreau

After three weeks, you might feel great and be sailing through your steps, or you might be beginning to feel it is a bit of a grind. If you fall into the latter category, have a look at the ideas on page 104 and see if you can get remotivated for another push.

- If you are a beginner, you should be aiming to do 5,600–6,700 steps each day this week.
- If you are an intermediate, or are aiming for weight loss, try for 6,800–7,900 steps each day this week.
- If you consider yourself fairly fit, try to do at least 7,900 steps each day this week.

If you are getting on well with your step targets, it may be interesting to try a 10,000-step day. See how it feels and how easy it is to complete the total. If you are struggling for time in your daily step count, now is the time to begin upping the pace and trying to do a few more steps in each walk you take.

Anyone trying to lose weight should now be sticking as much as possible to the recommendations in Chapter 8. Your steps are reaching the point where they should begin to have an impact in the form of weight loss and it would be a shame to walk all that way just to spoil it by cheating on your food.

Monday

Date: ....

Step target: ....

Steps walked: ....

Weekly total so far: ....

Intensity: ....

Calorie intake: ....

Calories burned: ....

Notes: ....

....

....

.

Tuesday

Date: ....

Step target: ....

Steps walked: ....

Weekly total so far: ....

Intensity: ....

Calorie intake: ....

Calories burned: ....

Notes: ....
....
....

Wednesday

Date: ....

Step target: ....

Steps walked: ....

Weekly total so far: ....

Intensity: ....

Calorie intake: ....

Calories burned: ....

Notes: ....
....
....

Thought for the day

THE FIRST WEALTH IS HEALTH

— Ralph Waldo Emerson

Thursday

Date: ....

Step target: ....

Steps walked: ....

Weekly total so far: ....

Intensity: ....

Calorie intake: ....

Calories burned: ....

Notes: ....

....

....

Thought for the day

WE DO NOT STOP PLAYING BECAUSE WE
GROW OLD; WE GROW OLD BECAUSE WE
STOP PLAYING – Anon

Friday

Date: ....

Step target: ....

Steps walked: ....

Weekly total so far: ....

Intensity: ....

Calorie intake: ....

Calories burned: ....

Notes: ....

....

....

Thought for the day

EVERY BATTLE IS WON BEFORE IT IS
FOUGHT – Sun Tzu, The Art of War

Saturday

Date: ....

Step target: ....

Steps walked: ....

Weekly total so far: ....

Intensity: ....

Calorie intake: ....

Calories burned: ....

Notes: ....

....

....

Thought for the day

TO IMPROVE IS TO CHANGE. TO BE
PERFECT IS TO CHANGE OFTEN
– Winston Churchill

Sunday

Date: ....

Step target: ....

Steps walked: ....

Weekly total so far: ....

Intensity: ....

Calorie intake: ....

Calories burned: ....

Notes: ....

....

....

Thought for the day

SUCCESS SEEMS TO BE LARGELY A
MATTER OF HANGING ON AFTER
OTHERS HAVE LET GO – William Feather

Week Five

Thought for the week

HAPPY IS THE MAN WHO HAS ACQUIRED
THE LOVE OF WALKING FOR ITS OWN
SAKE! – W J Holland

Congratulations! You have stuck it out for a month.
Hopefully, walking is becoming much more routine for you
now. Have you noticed how much more time you have to
think? Holiday plans, work problems, relationship issues –
your long walk is the perfect opportunity to sift things
through in your mind.

- If you are a beginner, you should be aiming to do
  6,300–7,400 steps each day this week.
- If you are an intermediate, or are aiming for weight loss,
  try for 7,500–8,500 steps each day this week.
- If you consider yourself fairly fit, try to do at least 8,600
  steps each day this week.

In the intensity space on your chart, you can now start trying
to chart accurately the exertions of your major walk or walks
of the day. Try to determine how much time you spent in
each zone so you can refer to this as you try to get more
from your walk.

Those attempting to lose weight should remember to
restrict the size of portions. Even foods you think are not
full of calories can build you up if you eat too much of
them. And, don't feel bad about throwing away leftovers;
if you don't want it, you don't need it.

Monday

Date: ....

Step target: ....

Steps walked: ....

Weekly total so far: ....

Intensity: ....

Calorie intake: ....

Calories burned: ....

Notes: ....
....
....

Thought for the day

HE THAT FIGHTS AND RUNS AWAY LIVES
TO FIGHT ANOTHER DAY – Anon

Tuesday

Date: ....

Step target: ....

Steps walked: ....

Weekly total so far: ....

Intensity: ....

Calorie intake: ....

Calories burned: ....

Notes: ....

....

....

Thought for the day

FAILURE IS THE OPPORTUNITY TO
BEGIN AGAIN MORE EFFICIENTLY
– Henry Ford

Wednesday

Date: ....

Step target: ....

Steps walked: ....

Weekly total so far: ....

Intensity: ....

Calorie intake: ....

Calories burned: ....

Notes: ....
....
....

Thought for the day

I HAVE TWO DOCTORS: MY LEFT LEG

AND MY RIGHT – G M Trevelyan

Thursday

Date: ....

Step target: ....

Steps walked: ....

Weekly total so far: ....

Intensity: ....

Calorie intake: ....

Calories burned: ....

Notes: ....

....

....

Friday

Date: ....

Step target: ....

Steps walked: ....

Weekly total so far: ....

Intensity: ....

Calorie intake: ....

Calories burned: ....

Notes: ....
....
....

Thought for the day

HOW MANY ROADS MUST A MAN WALK
DOWN, BEFORE YOU CALL HIM A MAN?
– Bob Dylan, 'Blowing in the Wind'

Saturday

Date: ....

Step target: ....

Steps walked: ....

Weekly total so far: ....

Intensity: ....

Calorie intake: ....

Calories burned: ....

Notes: ....

....

....

Thought for the day

OH! HOW I HATE TO GET UP IN THE
MORNING. OH! HOW I'D LOVE TO
REMAIN IN BED – Irving Berlin

Sunday

Date: ....

Step target: ....

Steps walked: ....

Weekly total so far: ....

Intensity: ....

Calorie intake: ....

Calories burned: ....

Notes: ....

....

....

Thought for the day

KEEP RIGHT ON TO THE END OF THE
ROAD, KEEP RIGHT ON TO THE END
– Sir Harry Lauder (song)

Week Six

Thought for the week

IF ONE JUST KEEPS ON WALKING,
EVERYTHING WILL BE ALL RIGHT
– Soren Kierkegaard

OK, things are going to get tougher now. Not only are you approaching your goal of 10,000 steps, but you should also be looking to walk about a third of your target at a pace that will leave you puffing when you finish.

- If you are a beginner, you should be aiming to do 7,000–8,100 steps each day this week.
- If you are an intermediate, or are aiming for weight loss, try for 8,200–9,300 steps each day this week.
- If you consider yourself fairly fit, try to do at least 9,400 steps each day this week.

Are you still creating new challenges for your walks? If you haven't already, now is the time to begin tackling a few hills. Start timing how long it takes you to reach the peak of the hill and take notice of how tackling a hill at pace affects you. It will take a lot more out of you.

If your strict diet is taking its toll on your morale, allow yourself a day off. Plan it ahead so you don't feel you have lost control, and think of it as part of the programme not as a failure.

Monday

Date: . . . .

Step target: . . . .

Steps walked: . . . .

Weekly total so far: . . . .

Intensity: . . . .

Calorie intake: . . . .

Calories burned: . . . .

Notes: . . . .

. . . .

. . . .

Thought for the day

PROCRASTINATION IS THE THIEF OF
TIME – Edward Young

Tuesday

Date: ....

Step target: ....

Steps walked: ....

Weekly total so far: ....

Intensity: ....

Calorie intake: ....

Calories burned: ....

Notes: ....

....

....

Thought for the day

FOOTFALLS ECHO IN THE MEMORY
DOWN THE PASSAGE WHICH WE DID
NOT TAKE – T S Eliot

Wednesday

Date: ....

Step target: ....

Steps walked: ....

Weekly total so far: ....

Intensity: ....

Calorie intake: ....

Calories burned: ....

Notes: ....

....

....

Thought for the day

LIFE IS ONE LONG PROCESS OF GETTING TIRED – Samuel Butler

Thursday

Date: ....

Step target: ....

Steps walked: ....

Weekly total so far: ....

Intensity: ....

Calorie intake: ....

Calories burned: ....

Notes: ....

....

....

Thought for the day

THE GOLDEN RULE IS THAT THERE ARE
NO GOLDEN RULES – *George Bernard Shaw*

Friday

Date: . . . .

Step target: . . . .

Steps walked: . . . .

Weekly total so far: . . . .

Intensity: . . . .

Calorie intake: . . . .

Calories burned: . . . .

Notes: . . . .

. . . .

. . . .

Thought for the day

THE WOODS ARE LOVELY, DARK AND
DEEP, BUT I HAVE PROMISES TO KEEP.
AND MILES TO GO BEFORE I SLEEP
– Robert Frost

Saturday

Date: . . . .

Step target: . . . .

Steps walked: . . . .

Weekly total so far: . . . .

Intensity: . . . .

Calorie intake: . . . .

Calories burned: . . . .

Notes: . . . .

. . . .

. . . .

. . . .

Thought for the day

I FIND THE GREAT THING IN LIFE IS NOT
SO MUCH WHERE WE STAND, AS IN
WHAT DIRECTION WE ARE MOVING
– Oliver Wendell Holmes

Sunday

Date: ....

Step target: ....

Steps walked: ....

Weekly total so far: ....

Intensity: ....

Calorie intake: ....

Calories burned: ....

Notes: ....

....

....

Thought for the day

SUNDAY CLEARS AWAY THE RUST OF
THE WHOLE WEEK – Joseph Addison

Week Seven

EVERYWHERE IS IN WALKING DISTANCE

IF YOU HAVE THE TIME – Steven Wright

Many of you will be reaching the magic figure of
10,000 steps this week. Hopefully, as it is getting easier
and easier, you are working harder and harder.
Ten thousand steps will help you maintain a healthy
lifestyle, but it is how you do them that will determine
whether your fitness and weight will improve.

- If you are a beginner, you should be aiming to do
  7,800–9,000 steps each day this week.
- If you are an intermediate, or are aiming for weight
  loss, try for 9,000–10,000 steps each day this week.
- If you consider yourself fairly fit, try to do at least
  10,000 steps each day this week.

When you are exercising rigorously, concentrate on
your breathing. Breathe in through your nose, letting
your stomach rise up and let your lungs fill with as
much air as you can. When you breathe out, take it
steady, releasing the air from your stomach up through
your mouth.

  If you are not losing weight by now, it is likely you
are taking your walking too lightly. Step up the pace
and you should start seeing some results.

Monday

Date: ....

Step target: ....

Steps walked: ....

Weekly total so far: ....

Intensity: ....

Calorie intake: ....

Calories burned: ....

Notes: ....

....

....

Thought for the day

FAR AWAY IS CLOSE AT HAND

– Robert Graves

Tuesday

Date: . . . .

Step target: . . . .

Steps walked: . . . .

Weekly total so far: . . . .

Intensity: . . . .

Calorie intake: . . . .

Calories burned: . . . .

Notes: . . . .

. . . .

. . . .

Thought for the day

THE JOURNEY OF A THOUSAND MILES BEGINS WITH A SINGLE STEP – Lau Tzu

Wednesday

Date: ....

Step target: ....

Steps walked: ....

Weekly total so far: ....

Intensity: ....

Calorie intake: ....

Calories burned: ....

Notes: ....

....

....

Thought for the day

SO MANY PATHS THAT WIND AND WIND

– Ella Wheeler Wilcox

Thursday

Date: ....

Step target: ....

Steps walked: ....

Weekly total so far: ....

Intensity: ....

Calorie intake: ....

Calories burned: ....

Notes: ....
....
....

Thought for the day

CLIMB EV'RY MOUNTAIN, FORD EV'RY
STREAM FOLLOW EV'RY RAINBOW,
'TILL YOU FIND YOUR DREAM
– Oscar Hammerstein II

Friday

Date: ....

Step target: ....

Steps walked: ....

Weekly total so far: ....

Intensity: ....

Calorie intake: ....

Calories burned: ....

Notes: ....

....

....

Thought for the day

THE POETRY OF MOTION

– Kenneth Grahame

Saturday

Date: ....

Step target: ....

Steps walked: ....

Weekly total so far: ....

Intensity: ....

Calorie intake: ....

Calories burned: ....

Notes: ....

....

....

Thought for the day

IT'S ONLY A STEP FROM THE SUBLIME

TO THE RIDICULOUS

– Napoleon Bonaparte

Sunday

Date: ....

Step target: ....

Steps walked: ....

Weekly total so far: ....

Intensity: ....

Calorie intake: ....

Calories burned: ....

Notes: ....
....
....

Thought for the day

IT IS GOOD TO BE OUT ON THE ROAD,
AND GOING ONE KNOWS NOT WHERE
– John Masefield

Week Eight

Thought for the week

MY GRANDMOTHER STARTED WALKING FIVE MILES A DAY WHEN SHE WAS 60. SHE'S 93 TODAY AND WE DON'T KNOW WHERE THE HELL SHE IS.

– Ellen DeGeneres

You should all be at, or approaching, 10,000 steps a day. It might have been hard work, but now you are there, don't stop. Keep it going and the benefits should be just around the corner. Exactly what you choose to do is up to you. Many people will just want to keep it at that level and carry on improving their fitness; some will want to take it further (see Nordic Striding and Race Walking on pages 119 and 120) and, unfortunately, some will fall by the wayside – don't let that be you.

If you are trying to lose weight, it might be necessary for you to carry on past 10,000 and add more steps to your target. Remember not to increase your total by more than 10 per cent a week and, when you reach your target weight, you can feel OK about reducing your target to 10,000 steps again.

If you suddenly find the walks much more difficult, you could be overdoing it. Take a break for a day or two and refresh your batteries. When you restart, take it fairly easy for a couple of days before resuming your regime.

Well done and step on...

Monday

Date: ....

Step target: ....

Steps walked: ....

Weekly total so far: ....

Intensity: ....

Calorie intake: ....

Calories burned: ....

Notes: ....

....

....

Thought for the day

IF YOU CAN'T EXCEL WITH TALENT,

TRIUMPH WITH EFFORT – Weinbaum

Tuesday

Date: ....

Step target: ....

Steps walked: ....

Weekly total so far: ....

Intensity: ....

Calorie intake: ....

Calories burned: ....

Notes: ....

....

....

Thought for the day

WHAT WOULD LIFE BE IF WE HAD NO
COURAGE TO ATTEMPT ANYTHING?
– Vincent van Gogh

Wednesday

Date: ....

Step target: ....

Steps walked: ....

Weekly total so far: ....

Intensity: ....

Calorie intake: ....

Calories burned: ....

Notes: ....

....

....

Thought for the day

THERE IS NO SUCH THING IN ANYONE'S
LIFE AS AN UNIMPORTANT DAY
– Alexander Woolcott

Thursday

Date: ....

Step target: ....

Steps walked: ....

Weekly total so far: ....

Intensity: ....

Calorie intake: ....

Calories burned: ....

Notes: ....
....
....

Thought for the day

IF YOU THINK YOU CAN, YOU CAN. AND
IF YOU THINK YOU CAN'T YOU'RE RIGHT
— Mary Kay Ash

Friday

Date: ....

Step target: ....

Steps walked: ....

Weekly total so far: ....

Intensity: ....

Calorie intake: ....

Calories burned: ....

Notes: ....
....
....

Thought for the day

RESPECT YOURSELF MOST OF ALL

– Pythagaros

Saturday

Date: ....

Step target: ....

Steps walked: ....

Weekly total so far: ....

Intensity: ....

Calorie intake: ....

Calories burned: ....

Notes: ....

....

....

Thought for the day

YOU KNOW MORE THAN YOU THINK
YOU DO – Dr Spock

Sunday

Date: ....

Step target: ....

Steps walked: ....

Weekly total so far: ....

Intensity: ....

Calorie intake: ....

Calories burned: ....

Notes: ....
....
....

Thought for the day

WHAT WAS HARD TO BEAR IS SWEET TO
REMEMBER – Portuguese proverb